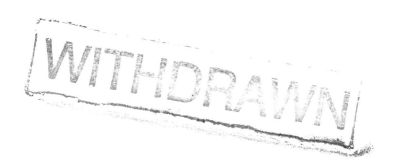

THE CAESAREAN

Today, in many parts of the world, at least one baby in four is born by caesarean. This is the first book that addresses all the key issues related to the procedure.

Having been involved as a participant in half a century of the history of the caesarean, Dr Michel Odent is uniquely equipped to authoritatively raise these vital and urgent questions.

- How did a magnificent rescue operation become such a common way of being born?
- Why is the rate 10 per cent or less in some places, and 50 per cent or more in other places?
- Why have risky procedures, such as forceps delivery, not been eliminated by the caesarean?
- Why should we take a different approach to non-labour caesareans, labour caesareans and emergency caesareans?
- What is the birthing pool test?
- What are the very first microbes met by a caesarean born baby?
- Is it easy to breastfeed after a caesarean?
- What do we know about the long-term consequences of being born by caesarean?
- What do we know about the long-term consequences of giving birth by caesarean?
- What do mother and her baby miss out on by not having a vaginal birth?
- How did the caesarean become safer and safer?
- What is the future of à la carte scheduled C-section?
- Is the age of the caesarean a landmark in the evolution of brain size?
- Are we moving towards an unprecedented cultural diversity?
- What is the future of a civilization born by caesarean?

Can humanity survive the safe caesarean?

THE CAESAREAN

Michel Odent

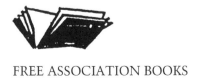

FREE ASSOCIATION BOOKS

First published in Great Britain 2004 by
FREE ASSOCIATION BOOKS
One Angel Cottages, Milespit Hill, London NW7 1RD

www.fabooks.com

A catalogue record for this book is available from the British Library

ISBN 978 1 85343 718 2 hbk

This book is made from paper suitable for recycling and made from fully
managed and sustained forest sources. Logging, pulping and manufacturing
processes are expected to conform to the environmental standards of the
country of origin.

10   9   8   7   6   5   4   3

Produced for Free Association Books by Chase Publishing Services Ltd
Printed and bound in the European Union by
CPI Antony Rowe, Chippenham and Eastbourne, England

CONTENTS

ACKNOWLEDGMENTS

I owe a special debt to the midwives and surgical nurses of the Pithiviers hospital, with whom I shared the experience of about one thousand 'in-labour caesareans' … during all hours of day and night.

This book greatly benefited from the constant constructive criticism of Sylvie Donna, and from conversations and correspondence with Jane English, the author of *Different Doorway*.

Special thanks to Liliana Lammers, for her encouragement and her enthusiasm.

1 A MAGNIFICENT RESCUE OPERATION

Between November 1953 and April 1954 I spent half a year in the maternity unit of a Paris hospital as an 'extern'. At that time an extern was a selected medical student with minor clinical responsibilities. I did this period of training in obstetrics by chance, just because a post was vacant. As I had no special interest in childbirth and no intention of becoming an obstetrician, and also because I needed time to prepare intensively for important exams, I spent as little time as possible in the maternity unit. However, it was long enough to learn the basics of obstetrics and to realize that the history of childbirth was entering a new phase.

MY COMMENTS AS AN OBSERVER

I often claim that, after participating in a conference, I usually just remember what I learnt in the corridors or in the restaurant. I might say the same about what I learnt in the departments of certain hospitals. Once I had lunch with one of the interns of this maternity unit where I was an extern. In the 1950s an intern in a Paris hospital was a selected junior doctor with vital responsibilities. During our conversation about the fast evolution of medicine since the Second World War, he told me his vision of the future of obstetrics. 'The practice of obstetrics will be so simple', he said. 'If the birth is easy and straightforward the vaginal route will be considered possible. If it is long and difficult there will be no reason for procrastination. It will be easy to do a low-segmental caesarean section'. 'Low segmental' is the technical term to qualify the new safe technique that was gradually spreading in the 1950s. During my half-year as an extern I was given one opportunity to scrub and participate in a low-segmental section. That was enough to understand the main steps of the operation. The rate of C-sections at that time in that unit probably was in the region of 1 per cent.

There were major obstacles to developing the new technique. The main one was that very few doctors involved in childbirth had a surgical background. Most of them were dependent on surgeons who had not yet learnt the new technique. They had a deep-rooted attachment to the forceps, which for three centuries had been the symbol of obstetrical practice. The informal conversation I had at lunchtime with the clever intern probably helped me to realize that many doctors preferred to ignore the advent of the safe technique of the C-section, as if they felt threatened by the surgeons and their prestigious status. The fact that I was an observer and an outsider in this obstetrical milieu, since I had already decided to become a surgeon, helped me to perceive the semi-conscious motivations of different practitioners, according to their age and their background. I find it significant in retrospect that the head of the maternity unit – who gave his name to forceps – was intriguingly silent on the topic of caesareans. I never heard him making any allusion to its future.

MY COMMENTS AS AN ACTOR

As soon as I became an intern I did all my training in surgical units because from the very beginning of my medical studies I had decided to become a surgeon. My need to be useful and efficient could not be met in medical units, performing diagnoses. (Since we were immersed in hospital activities from the very first day of our medical studies, it was easy for me to decide this.) I noticed that brilliant doctors who discussed sophisticated diagnoses had a disdain for therapeutics and were unable to influence the evolution of a disease, more often than not. Surgery was different, though. I could not forget one of the first patients I saw in a surgical unit with a strangulated hernia. A simple emergency operation saved her life.

Once when I was on duty at night in the surgical unit, it just so happened that a friend from the maternity unit called me to help him with an emergency caesarean. This is how I learnt the new technique. I could not have guessed that occasionally helping a friend in the middle of the night might one day give my career a new direction.

Then, from 1958 to 1959, I was doing my military service in the war of independence in Algeria. I spent most of my time in the army at the hospital of Tizi-Ouzou, the main city of the Kabylia region, in the Berber part of Algeria. We were busy both day and night, performing all sorts of emergency surgery, mostly war-related. Now and then, a woman would arrive from a mountain village with a protracted labour. By doing a low-segmental caesarean, I was in a position to rescue the baby. The day after the emergency operation, the whole village was aware of what was seen as a miracle. Later, in the summer of 1960, I covered for a surgeon in Guinea, West Africa ... which was another opportunity to introduce the safe technique.

In 1962 I learnt that a hospital 50 miles from Paris needed to recruit a doctor to be in charge of its surgical unit. I applied for the post without even visiting the hospital. I wanted to be outside Paris without being too far away. This is how I came to move to Pithiviers. Close to the surgical unit and in the same building there was a small maternity unit with two midwives who enthusiastically welcomed me when they heard that I could do the safe modern technique of C-section. There was an older surgeon locally who was still doing the classical operation. The first time I did a C-section in Pithiviers, between a hernia repair and a gallbladder operation, I heard the senior surgical nurse exclaiming: 'What a magnificent rescue operation!'

2   ONE ROUTE OR THE OTHER

A GLOBAL PHENOMENON

At the dawn of the twenty-first century, the granddaughters of women who gave birth when I was a medical student usually regard the caesarean in a 'modern' way. For most of them it is just one of the two routes a baby can enter the world. Today, in certain places, it is even the most common way of being born. It has become a consumer good. In Brazil, this huge country whose population equals the total of the German, French and Spanish populations, the overall rate of C-sections is well above 50 per cent. Of course there are differences between cities and rural areas, and also between private and public hospitals: in the private hospitals of big cities such as São Paulo and Rio, four out of five babies are born by caesarean – 80 per cent! In some clinics, the policy is to perform a caesarean unless the woman requests otherwise. A pro-caesarean culture is spreading. Fear of substandard care is behind many poor women's preference for a caesarean.[1] In Brazilian public hospitals, 'only' 40 per cent of babies are born by caesarean. Practices and statistics are similar in other large Latin American cities, such as Mexico City or Santiago, and in the southern half of Italy.

If the current trend continues, it is likely that in the near future many cities and even countries all over the world will also pass the 50 per cent mark. This long list includes a great part of the Asian continent: India (particularly Delhi), the whole of China, Taiwan, Thailand, Singapore, South Korea, and it includes the majority of Latin America (including Cuba but not Bolivia). Turkey (in particular Istanbul), Greece, Spain and Portugal might also join the list. Even in countries that are not included in this list, the caesarean is now considered a common way of being born. In the US, for example, about 26 per cent of babies are born by caesarean. In most Western and continental European countries, such as the UK, France, Germany, Switzerland, Hungary, and also in Australia and New Zealand, at least one in five babies has a caesarean birth.

THE RIGHT TO CHOOSE

As soon as the caesarean was perceived as a common way to give birth, the right to choose became acceptable and we entered the age of caesarean section on demand. From 1997 onwards, the issue has been repeatedly discussed in authoritative medical journals.[2,3,4,5] The new phenomenon of elective caesarean on demand originally developed in Italy and in the largest Latin American cities before spreading all over the world. At the end of the twentieth century, doctors were wondering if they would accept performing a section on demand.[4] At the beginning of the twenty-first century, they wonder if all women should be offered an elective caesarean delivery.[6] There is a constant increase in the rates of patient-choice caesareans. In the US, these rates went from 1.56 per cent of all deliveries in 1999 to 1.87 per cent in 2001.

Certain obstetricians are directly or indirectly participating in the rapid development of these new tendencies. Interestingly, in a survey of obstetricians' preference, 31 per cent of London female obstetricians with an uncomplicated pregnancy at term claimed that they would choose a scheduled caesarean delivery for themselves.[7] Similar preferences have been expressed among female and male North American obstetricians.[8] Professor Steer, an influential professor of obstetrics in London, suggests theoretical considerations to support the new attitudes; he underlined that the human brain size represents the main challenge to the birth process, and he considers the caesarean section to be an 'evolving procedure', that is a technological solution to 'the conflict between the need to think and the need to run'.[9] He anticipates that in the future the unpredictable risks of labour will no longer be justified for most women. If caesarean section does become the norm, average birth weight will no longer be restricted by the constraints of maternal pelvic size so that eventually caesarean birth will become necessary for the majority.

Comparable opinions are expressed on both sides of the Atlantic. The American College of Obstetricians and Gynecologists' ethics committee published in October 2003 a statement judging elective caesareans ethical. W. Benson Harer Jr, medical director of the Riverside County Regional Medical Center in Moreno Valley, California, commented on this statement: 'I think it is a step to where we're going. And my guess is that as increasing evidence comes out, it will probably become a more accepted procedure.'[10] At the same time, in the UK, the National Institute for Clinical Excellence (NICE) issued preliminary guidelines making clear that doctors should not refuse a woman the right to have a caesarean, but that the reasons for the request should be sought, recorded and discussed. In the countries where access to health care is socialized there will be a tendency to avoid the additional cost of an acceptance of all maternal requests.

'Birth from above' or 'birth from below'? Such an unprecedented choice offered to the new generations is undoubtedly a landmark in the history of ... mammals. Within a few decades a rescue operation has become a common way of being born. How has this happened?

3   SAFER AND SAFER

The main reason why caesarean rates have risen almost everywhere in the world is that this operation has become safe.

THE INDIRECT VERSUS THE DIRECT ROUTE

In terms of safety the turning point came soon after the Second World War, when the new technique started to spread. Before then the most direct route was used to open the uterus. The skin, the fascias and the uterine muscle were cut by vertical (up and down) incisions from about an inch above the navel to about an inch above the pubic bone. For many reasons this classical section was done as a last resort. The risks of bleeding from the thick uterine wall and the risks of infection were too high; bowel adhesions to the uterine scar could cause intestinal obstruction; healing of the uterine muscle was often faulty and the risk of bloody scar rupture in subsequent pregnancies was in the region of 2 per cent.

The principle of the new technique was to open the uterine muscle by a transverse (side to side) incision at a different place: a thin zone called the low segment. The cervix of the uterus is divided into a vaginal part and an intra-abdominal part. The intra-abdominal part develops at the end of the pregnancy and becomes the low segment. It is covered by a mobile sheet of peritoneum (the mucous membrane that covers the abdominal organs). The risks of all sorts of complications were dramatically reduced with the low-segmental technique. This occurred at the very time when safer methods of anaesthesia were developing, when the first antibiotics were available, when blood transfusion became possible and when the replacement of gum pipes by plastic pipes made intravenous drips much safer. So, for a combination of reasons, a last-resort, risky operation became a safe operation in the space of a few years.

The caesarean technique that is in use today is not fundamentally different from the one that was developed in the 1950s. I must emphasise the word 'developed', because several obstetricians had experimented in the past with transverse incisions into the lower segment of the uterus. This indirect route had been advocated in the early twentieth century by Munro Kerr,[1] a professor of midwifery at the University of Glasgow, and promulgated by influential American obstetricians such as Joseph DeLee. But it was in the 1950s that the new technique started to routinely supersede the old one all over the world.

PFANNENSTIEL AND THE BIKINI REVOLUTION

Since that time a series of improvements have made the caesarean even more acceptable and still safer. Up to the late 1960s, the skin incision – the visible part of the operation – remained the same, that is to say vertical from the navel to the pubic bone. It was easy, fast and safe. This sort of incision of the abdominal wall was acceptable as long as the caesarean was understood as a rare rescue operation, although the skin scar of a vertical incision occasionally remains thick, large and red. When 'birth from above' became commonplace, aesthetic considerations had to be taken into account especially since, on the beach, this was the time of the bikini revolution.

As early as 1900, Hermann Pfannenstiel, a surgeon and gynaecologist from Breslau, Germany, had described a side-to-side incision just above the pubic hair.[2] Soon after, the Pfannenstiel incision was mentioned in all textbooks on surgical technique and used by many surgeons for various gynaecological operations. However, for a long time very few practitioners thought of using this route for delivering a baby. Even if they were already familiar with the incision, they considered it inappropriate for a caesarean. The first reason for this reluctance was the need to be as fast as possible. We must keep in mind that for several decades one of the preoccupations of most surgeons was that the drugs used for the general anaesthesia would not have the time to reach the baby. There was a sort of race between the surgeon reaching the baby and the drug reaching the placenta. In fact there was another semi-conscious reason that I probably shared with many others in the 1960s. We could not easily imagine a big baby getting out through a small side-to-side incision in the pubic hair. It is in the late 1960s that I personally dared to try this route for a caesarean. After performing half a dozen caesareans that way, I realized that I was almost as fast as with the more familiar vertical skin incision. Without my knowing it, a nurse recorded that I took two minutes and ten seconds between the skin incision and the birth of the baby. Women started to compare their tiny almost invisible scar in the pubic hair with occasionally ugly vertical scars. And the C-section became more acceptable than ever.

THE AGE OF EPIDURALS

Since the 1980s there has been a constant interaction between progress in the organization of hospitals and health professions on the one hand, and technical advances on the other.

This interaction is illustrated by the history of epidural anaesthesia. The concept of regional nerve blocks in general and of the epidural block in particular is not new. What is new is the popularity of the epidural block in childbirth. The anaesthetic drug is administered through a fine tube inserted through a needle in the woman's back (after a local anaesthetic has numbed the area) into a space between the spinal cord and the outer membrane. After 1980 demand for this procedure increased dramatically, so more and more anaesthesiologists became familiar with the use of this technique in obstetrics. The popularity of the epidural in childbirth therefore led to the advent of obstetric anaesthesiology, a sort of sub-specialty. The daily use of epidural anaesthesia during labour in certain maternity units created new situations. When a caesarean was decided upon, many women were already under the effect of the epidural. The advantages of a regional block over general anaesthesia appeared obvious, in that the mother was awake during the caesarean and was alert afterwards.

The development of obstetric anaesthesiology was, in turn, at the root of technical advances. In a conventional epidural a local anaesthetic also numbs the nerves that control the muscles of the lower part of the body, so that the labouring woman usually cannot move her legs. This is the reason for recent forms of epidurals. The dose of local anaesthetic can be significantly reduced, when used in combination with a morphine-like drug such as fentanyl. This combination epidural has been popularized by the term 'walking epidural'. Another popular form of the epidural is the combined spinal-epidural, where a one-off dose of a morphine-like drug, with or without local anaesthetic, is injected into the spinal space, very close to the end of the spinal cord. This gives pain relief for around two hours, and if further pain relief is needed, it is given as an epidural. Because there are no blood vessels within the spinal cord, the drugs do not diffuse into the maternal bloodstream. Today, in the case of a scheduled caesarean, a spinal block is often used.

The main effect of such advances in anaesthesiology is that the caesarean section is more and more acceptable and safer.

SCALPEL OR FINGERS?

The technique of the caesarean section is still evolving. In the 1990s Michael Stark and the team at the Misgav Ladach Hospital in Jerusalem introduced a method based on the Joel-Cohen incision, which was originally used for the hysterectomy.[3] This method restricts the use of sharp instruments, preferring manual manipulation instead. One of the objectives is to remove every unnecessary step. It is worth explaining the particularities of this technique, so that the advantages, in terms of speed and blood loss, can be easily understood by health professionals and lay people as well.[4]

The skin incision is, as usual, horizontal above the pubic hair. The first difference from the usual technique is that the scalpel incision of the layer of fat under the skin is just an inch long on the midline, so that the lateral tissue is separated by stretching with two fingers. This is a way to avoid cutting small vessels. The same with the fascia covering the muscles, which is manually separated along its fibres. The muscles are separated by pulling. The peritoneum is opened by stretching with index fingers. The uterus is opened with an index finger and the hole enlarged between the index finger of one hand and the thumb of the other. After the delivery of the baby and of the placenta, the uterus may be lifted through the incision onto the draped abdominal wall. This makes the suture of the uterine muscle as safe as possible, with perfect visual control. After that only the fascia and the skin are stitched. It is well understood today that the peritoneum heals rapidly and more completely when it is not stitched.[5]

An accumulation of data confirms that this Michael Stark technique can reduce blood loss and operating time. For example, according to a Swedish evaluation, the average blood loss was 250 ml with the new technique versus 400 ml with the usual technique. As for the average operating time, it was 20 minutes, as compared with the usual technique's 28 minutes.[6] Another indication of how the caesarean is getting safer and safer. In the particular case of HIV-positive mothers, the priority is to protect the baby from the risk of transmission of the virus. An adapted technique is now promoted (the haemostatic caesarean technique) so that the baby is born perfectly clean, without any trace of maternal blood on its body.

CAN WE MEASURE THE SAFETY OF THE CAESAREAN?

In general, those who are directly involved in obstetrics regard the modern caesarean as a safe operation. It is significant that many women obstetricians choose to have a caesarean for the birth of their own babies. The point is that it is difficult to express the degree of safety in statistical language. The golden method in medical research in order to compare two possible treatments, or policies, or strategies, is based on randomization: this means that a population is first divided into groups after drawing lots. One group is allocated a treatment, while another group is allocated – at random – another treatment. Then, during a follow-up period, the comparative ratios of benefits to risks for both treatments are evaluated and expressed in statistical language. For obvious reasons one cannot tell a group of pregnant women that they must give birth vaginally, while other women – at random – are told that they must have a caesarean.

However, we can learn from randomized trials that were not originally designed to evaluate the frequency of maternal health problems. One is a famous trial involving 121 centres in 26 countries, designed to compare a policy of planned caesarean section with a policy of planned vaginal birth in the case of a breech presentation at term.[7] More than 2,000 women were involved in this trial. It appeared that the rates of serious maternal health problems were roughly the same in both groups. Similar conclusions can be drawn from a study whose objective was to compare planned caesarean versus vaginal delivery in the prevention of HIV transmission in a population of 436 pregnant women.[8]

These findings are reinforced by a large Danish study[9] looking in retrospect at the 15,441 Danish women who gave birth to a first baby in a breech position between 1982 and 1995. Among them, 7,503 had a planned caesarean, 5,575 had an emergency caesarean and 2,363 gave birth vaginally. Contrary to received ideas, the incidence of haemorrhage and anaemia after planned caesarean section (5.7 per cent) did not differ from that after vaginal delivery and was slightly lower than after emergency caesarean (7 per cent). The rate of thromboembolic complications was 0.1 per cent after caesarean. On the other hand the anal sphincter rupture, which is associated with a subsequent risk of anal incontinence, was 1.7 per cent after vaginal birth. It is commonplace to emphasize that all surgical procedures carry an inherent risk of injuries to organs not directly involved in the particular surgery. The risks must be put in perspective. In these series there were just a few cases of bladder injuries (0.1 per cent during planned caesarean and 0.2 per cent during emergency caesarean) and a bladder injury can be easily and immediately repaired. Such risks will be still lower with techniques that restrict the use of sharp instruments. In this series it has never been necessary to perform a caesarean-hysterectomy (to remove all or part of the uterus) to stop the bleeding. The risks of post-operative adhesions (and therefore the risks of intestinal obstruction long after) are also very low after the modern caesarean, particularly if no foreign material such as gauze has been introduced in the abdomen. In the near future it might become routine to instil specific substances in the peritoneum to prevent adhesion formation.

The risk of maternal death is also difficult to evaluate. Once more the studies cannot be randomized. In most statistics the risks of maternal deaths appear to be three to four times higher after a caesarean than after a birth by the vaginal route.[10] But the studies are hampered by the fact that the women having caesarean delivery have conditions, pregnancy complications and delivery complications that are themselves associated with increased maternal mortality. Furthermore, in developed countries, one needs to analyse the outcomes of at least 100,000 births to significantly evaluate the rates of maternal deaths (or pregnancy-related deaths). These considerations are based on recent studies conducted in wealthy countries. (The issues are different when considering the case of rural areas of developing countries, particularly in sub-Saharan Africa,[11,12] where the rates of maternal deaths after caesareans can be 100 times higher than in developed countries.)

Whatever the perspective, one can claim today that, in modern, well-equipped and well-organized hospitals of developed countries, the safety of the caesarean is comparable to the safety of the vaginal route.

4   BREAKING A VICIOUS CIRCLE

FORGOTTEN NEEDS

If the safety of the procedure is the *prerequisite* for the widespread use of the C-section, it is *not the primary reason* for the increasing rates of obstetrical intervention. The primary reason for the increasing rates of intervention certainly is a quasi-cultural and universal lack of understanding of the basic needs of women in labour. After thousands of years of culturally controlled childbirth, a century of industrialization of obstetrics, a proliferation of 'methods' of 'natural childbirth' (as if the words 'method' and 'natural' were compatible), and the advent of a safe technique that offers another option than the vaginal route, one can easily explain why these basic needs are forgotten.

One cannot rely on any cultural model in order to rediscover the needs of women in labour. In most societies we know about, the cultural milieu usually interferes with the physiological processes via birth attendants who are more often than not active, even invasive, and via the transmission of beliefs and rituals. For instance, in many societies there is the belief that a birth attendant must be there to cut the cord immediately, which is a way to protect the newborn baby against the 'dangerous' colostrum or other 'negative' effects of skin-to-skin and eye-to-eye contacts between the mother and her newborn.

That is why we need the language and the perspective of modern physiologists (scientists who study the body functions) to go back to our roots, to look into what is cross cultural and universal, and therefore to rediscover the basic needs of labouring women. This perspective can also help us to realize that the reasons commonly given to explain the current high rates of caesarean sections – electronic foetal monitoring, fear of litigation, lack of midwives, alterations in the role of the midwives, high rates of labour inductions, frequent use of epidurals, and different aspects of the industrialization of childbirth in general – are basically the consequences of a widespread lack of understanding of birth physiology. In return, the safety of the caesarean tends to reinforce a traditional lack of interest for birth physiology.

A REDISCOVERY

Let us break the vicious circle by visualizing a labouring woman from the perspective of a modern physiologist.

This leads us to *focus on the most active part of her body*, that is the glands secreting all the hormones involved in childbirth. These hormonal agents originate in old, primitive brain structures called the hypothalamus and the pituitary gland. In other words, if we visualize a labouring woman as a modern physiologist would, we visualize the deep, primitive part of her brain that is working hard and releasing a flow of hormones. Today we are also in a position to understand that when there are inhibitions – during the birth process or during any sort of sexual experience – such inhibitions originate in the 'new brain', the part of the brain which is highly developed among humans and which can be seen as the brain of the intellect, or the thinking brain. It is more appropriate to call it the new cortex or, rather, the neocortex.

The key for rediscovering the universal needs of women in

labour is to interpret a phenomenon which is well known to certain mothers and midwives who have experience of undisturbed birth. It is the fact that when a woman is giving birth by herself, without any medication, there is a time when she has an obvious tendency to cut herself off from our world, as if *going to another planet*. She dares to do what she would never dare to do in her daily social life, for example scream or swear. She can find herself in the most unexpected postures, making the most unexpected noises. This means that she is reducing the control by the neocortex. This reduction of neocortical activity is the most important aspect of birth physiology from a practical point of view. It leads us to understand that a labouring woman needs first to be protected from any sort of stimulation of her neocortex. This can be translated in terms of dos and don'ts:

DON'T STIMULATE THE NEOCORTEX
OF A LABOURING WOMAN!

From a practical point of view it is useful to explain what this means and to review the well-known factors that can stimulate the human neocortex:

- *Language*, particularly rational language is one such factor. When we communicate with language we process what we perceive with our neocortex. This implies, for example, that one of the main qualities of a birth attendant is her capacity to keep a low profile and to remain silent, to avoid in particular asking precise questions. Imagine a woman in hard labour, and already 'on another planet'. She dares to scream out; she dares to do things she would never do otherwise; she has forgotten about what she has been taught or read in books; she has lost her sense of time and then she finds herself in the unexpected position of having to respond to someone who wants to know at what time she had her last pee! Although it is apparently simple, it will probably take a long time to rediscover that a birth attendant must remain as silent as possible.

- *Bright light* is another factor that stimulates the human neocortex. Electroencephalographers know that the trace exploring brain activity can be influenced by visual stimulation. We usually close the curtains and switch off the lights when we want to reduce the activity of our intellect in order to go to sleep. This implies that, from a physiological perspective, a dim light should in general facilitate the birth process. It will also take a long time to convince many health professionals that this is a serious issue. It is noticeable that as soon as a labouring woman is 'on another planet' she is spontaneously driven towards postures that tend to protect her against all sorts of visual stimulation. For example she may be on all fours, as if praying. Apart from reducing back pain, this common posture has many positive effects, such as eliminating the main reason for foetal distress (no compression of the big vessels that run along the spine) and facilitating the rotation of the baby's body.

- A *feeling of being observed* is another type of neocortical stimulation. The physiological response to the presence of an observer has been scientifically studied. In fact, it is common knowledge that we all feel different when we know we are being observed. In other words, *privacy* is a factor that facilitates the reduction of neocortical control. It is ironic that all non-human mammals, whose neocortex is not as developed as ours, have a strategy for giving birth in privacy – those who are normally active during the night, like rats, tend to give birth during the day, and conversely others like horses who are active during the day tend to give birth at night. Wild goats give birth in the most inaccessible mountain areas. Our close relatives the chimpanzees also move away from the group. The importance of privacy implies, for example, that there is a difference between the attitude of a midwife staying in front of a woman in labour and watching her, and another one just sitting in a corner. It implies also that we should be reluctant to introduce any device that can be perceived as a way to observe, be it a video camera or an electronic foetal monitor.

- Any situation likely to trigger a release of hormones of the adrenaline family also tends to stimulate the neocortex and to inhibit the birth process as a result. When there is a possible danger, mammals need to be alert and attentive. This implies that a labouring woman first *needs to feel secure*. The need to feel secure explains why all over the world and down throughout the ages many women had a tendency to give birth close to their mother, or close to a substitute for their mother – an experienced mother or grandmother – in the framework of the extended family or in the framework of the community … a midwife. The midwife was originally a mother-figure. The mother is the prototype of the person with whom one feels secure, without feeling observed and judged.

WHAT IF?

If the basic needs of labouring women had been recognized half a century ago – when the modern caesarean operation became widely known – the history of childbirth would undoubtedly have taken another direction. The reason for midwifery would have been taken into consideration. The *midwives* would not have disappeared, either completely, as has happened in certain countries, or de facto in many other countries where they lost their autonomy and their specificity, becoming the prisoners of protocols. When comparing countries, or cities, or hospitals, it is possible to guess what the rates of caesareans are by comparing the number of obstetricians and the number of midwives. In countries where obstetricians far outnumber the midwives, the midwives have lost their autonomy and the rates of C-sections have skyrocketed. This is the case of countries as diverse as Brazil and many other Latin American countries, China, South Korea, Taiwan, Turkey, Southern Italy and Greece.

If the basic needs of labouring women had been understood, we would not already be the witnesses of the second or third generation of high-tech childbirth. The transmission from mother to daughter of the predisposition to operative delivery is well-documented. A study of all women who were born in Utah during 1947–57 and who subsequently gave birth in Utah between 1970 and 1991 revealed in particular that when a woman had a caesarean for 'failure to progress' her daughter has a risk of giving birth by caesarean multiplied by 6.[1] One can wonder if the capacity to give birth is not gradually depleted since the dawn of industrialized childbirth.

If the basic needs of labouring women had been understood, the history of childbirth would never have entered its electronic age. Around 1970, doctors would have been reluctant to record continuously on a graph the rhythm of the baby's heartbeat and the power of the uterine contractions via an electronic machine. They would have realized that the fact that a labouring woman knows her body functions are being continuously monitored tends to stimulate her neocortex, and to make the birth longer, more difficult, and therefore more dangerous, so that more babies have to be rescued by C-section. Interestingly, it is only when the electronic age of childbirth was well-established all over the world that a series of large trials confirmed that the only constant and significant effect on statistics of *electronic foetal monitoring* – compared with listening to the heartbeat now and then – is to increase the caesarean rate.

If the electronic age of childbirth had been bypassed thanks to a sane understanding of the nature of birth, it is probable that *fear of litigation* would not have become an obsession. In the 1970s many doctors and the media had a tendency to transmit the belief that, thanks to electronic methods of monitoring, all the risks of childbirth could be eliminated ... as if an involuntary process can be controlled and 'managed' as easily as the flight of a jet. Such a belief implies that at the origin of any accident – a handicap, a death, etc. – there is always a mistake or a lack of care, and therefore a culprit.

If the right questions had been raised some decades ago, today we would not be the prisoners of well-established doctrines. *If*, for example, the central preoccupation had been with ensuring that the labouring woman maintain for as long as possible a maximally low level of adrenaline, it would have been easy to anticipate that the presence of a male neocortex stimulated by a release of stress hormones might be risky. Today nobody would even dare to point out that the advent of the new doctrines relating to the *father's participation in birth* and a spectacular increase in the rate of caesareans occurred concurrently (except in rare countries such as Ireland, where both the father's participation and the increased caesarean rates were postponed until the late 1980s).

A RULE OF THUMB

Since a lack of understanding of the physiological processes is directly or indirectly at the root of skyrocketing caesarean rates, a simple rule of thumb appears as an appropriate aid to rediscovering the basic needs of labouring women. It can be summarized in one sentence: where labour, delivery and birth are concerned, *what is specifically human must be eliminated, while the mammalian needs must be met*. To eliminate what is specifically human implies that the first step should be to get rid of the aftermath of all the beliefs (inseparable from rituals) that, for millennia, have disturbed the physiological processes in all known cultural milieux. (Such beliefs probably conferred an evolutionary advantage at a certain phase of the history of humankind.) It also implies that the activity of the neocortex, that part of the brain whose huge development is a human trait, needs to be reduced. It also implies that language, which is specifically human, must be used with extreme caution.

To meet the mammalian needs means first to satisfy the need for privacy, since all mammals have a strategy not to feel observed when giving birth. It also means satisfying the need to feel secure: the female of a mammal in the jungle cannot give birth as long as there is a predator around. It is significant that when a labouring woman has complete privacy and feels secure, she often finds herself in typically mammalian postures, for example on all fours.

It is commonplace to claim that childbirth should be 'humanized'. In fact, insofar as the objective is to moderate the caesarean rates, the priority should be to *'mammalianize' childbirth*. In a sense childbirth needs to be *de-humanized*.

5   WHEN OUR DREAMS COME TRUE

Myths, legends, poems and narratives tell us about universal and cross-cultural human dreams. With the advent of twentieth-century technological advances some of these dreams suddenly came true. This is the case of the caesarean, which can be presented as the realization of a deep-rooted archetypal fantasy. Let us follow an uncharted route in order to offer a novel interpretation of what might be called the caesarean temptation, that is to say the temptation to make the caesarean the most common way to give birth.

FROM ASCLEPIUS TO THE BARBIE DOLL

Asclepius, the Greek god of medicine, was born when his father Apollo cut the abdomen of his beloved Coronis, after she had been executed for infidelity. Zeus tore his son, Dionysus, from the womb of his dead mistress, and transplanted him into his own thigh, from which the baby was subsequently delivered. Such legends are not particular to the Greek culture. Numerous references to caesarean appear in ancient Hindu, Egyptian, Persian and European folklore. Ancient Chinese etchings depict the procedure on apparently living women. In the Shahnama, the 'Epic of Kings', written around 1000, which tells the stories of heroes of pre-Islamic Iran, there is a detailed description of a 'birth from above': Zal, a legendary hero called 'the Lion', implored the fabulous bird Simurgh for the delivery of his beloved Rudabeh. Simurgh gave his instructions so that the priest Mobed could cut the flank of Rudabeh with a dagger. This is how Rustam was miraculously born. It is noticeable that in all these ancient legends the operation was performed by a man, although childbirth was in general 'women business'.

In Germanic lore it was Tristan (in the version by Eilhart) who was born that way. One of the most striking images is that of the Antichrist's birth by caesarean in late medieval German woodcuts.

'Birth from above' was not foreign from the ancient British myths and folklores, as confirmed by this verse related to Macbeth's tragic downfall:

Despair thy charm;
And let the angel whom thou still hast serv'd
Tell thee, Macduff was from his mother's womb
Untimely ripp'd. (Act 5, scene 10)

Among the most picturesque legendary caesareans, one should mention those performed by the mother herself, and those performed by … the horns of a bull. The Frenchman Sacombe told in verse the story of a furious bull, in San Sebastian, who opened the tummy of a pregnant woman in such a way that the baby was born alive without going through the pelvis:

Le foetus sort vivant, sans franchir le pelvis.
[The foetus came out alive, without crossing the pelvis.]

It is hard to separate myths, legends, fiction and deception on the one hand, and historically verifiable facts on the other hand. The main reason for such difficulties is that in many societies the body of a dead pregnant woman could not be buried until the child had been removed. This is probably how a live baby was occasionally removed from a dying woman. In the eighth century BC, the Roman ruler Numa Pompillus passed a law requiring all women who died in labour to have a post-mortem delivery. This law continued throughout the reign of the Roman emperors, and was known as Lex Caesarea – *caesere* being the latin verb for 'to cut', a likely root for the term. The caesarean section operation did not derive its name from the fact that Julius Caesar was born in this manner. Julius Caesar could not have been born by Caesarean section, because his mother, Aurelia, lived to be an adviser to her grown son. It is possible that an ancestor of Caesar was named after surviving the surgical birth, and the name was passed down in the family. Later on the Catholic religion established a rule similar to the Lex Caesarea, in order to baptize the baby.

The caesarean was reserved for the tragic event of maternal death in labour, until the 1500s when the first operation was performed which resulted in the survival of both mother and baby. A Swiss swine-gelder, Jacques Nufer, offered to try performing a caesarean because his wife was suffering from a difficult obstructed labour, while 13 midwives and some lithotomists (surgeons extracting bladder stones) were present but could not give any useful advice. With a knife, in one go, he delivered an intact live baby. He stitched the wound and the mother recovered. This case was reported in the first treatise about caesareans on living women. Its authenticity was questioned by established physicians, because Mrs Nufer lived long enough to fire out six more children in the more traditional way, including a set of twins. One of the most plausible interpretations is that the foetus had developed outside the uterus (it might have been a so-called abdominal pregnancy). It is noticeable that the original text in Latin only mentions the incision of the abdominal wall, but is silent on the incision of the uterus. According to this interpretation, it was not a real caesarean.

Today, since the caesarean is such a safe and banal

intervention, one might think that our ancient dreams and fantasies are becoming extinct. Not so. There is a constant and irresistible resurgence of the most archetypal human fantasies. The success of the pregnant Barbie doll whose tummy can be opened is a highly significant example.

FROM ICARUS TO THE CROSS-CHANNEL GLIDER

Opening the tummy of a pregnant woman is not the only deep-rooted dream that came true in the most recent phases of the history of humankind. An analogy with another such ancient dream is not inopportune in order to support and clarify our interpretation of the caesarean temptation.

Icarus was imprisoned, with his father Daedalus, in a tower on Crete. They contrived to escape from their prison, but could not leave the island by sea as the king kept strict watch on all vessels. So they thought of escaping by air. Daedalus made wings with feathers for himself and for his young son. Daedalus arrived safe in Sicily, where he built a temple to Apollo and hung up his wings, as an offering to the god. But Icarus, exulting in his career, began to leave the guidance of his father and soar upward as if to reach heaven. The nearness of the blazing sun softened the wax which held the feathers together, and they came off. He fluttered with his arms, but no feathers remained to hold the air. While his mouth uttered cries to his father, it was submerged in the blue waters of the sea.

Bellerophon's greatest desire was to ride the magnificent winged flying horse, Pegasus. One day he woke to find a golden bridle at his feet. He went to Pegasus' favorite meadow and found the wonderful horse. Pegasus trotted right over and allowed himself to be mounted without a struggle. Unfortunately for Bellerophon, he was determined to become a god. One day, he urged Pegasus to fly toward Olympus, the home of the gods. Pegasus was wiser and for the first time, would not obey. He threw his rider to the ground and flew away.

These well-known legends are not particular to the Greek culture. There are many descriptions of flying machines and airborne beings in early Chinese, Korean and Indian texts. In the Vedic literature of India, the flying machines are usually called *vimanas*. Some are manmade craft that resemble airplanes and fly with the aid of birdlike wings. Others are unstreamlined structures that fly in a mysterious manner and are generally not made by human beings. Taoist tales often tell of adepts or immortals flying through the air. The Xian were immortals capable of flight under their own divine power. They were said to be feathered, and a term that has been used for Taoist priests is *yu ke*, meaning 'feathered guest'. The *fei tian*, which might be translated as 'flying immortals', also appear in early tales, adding to the numbers of airborne beings in the Chinese mythological corpus.

Today, at a time when flying from one continent to another is not an adventure, one might once more anticipate that some of the most archaic and universal of our dreams are becoming extinct. In fact the development and the popularity of a great variety of sports such as parachuting, skydiving, bungee jumping, paragliding, paramotoring and hang gliding are reminders of one of humankind's oldest dreams: personal flight. Glide across the Channel on carbon-fibre wings and you'll stimulate the Icarus dream among millions of your fellow creatures.

The caesarean temptation cannot be interpreted without referring to the mysterious universality of a small number of human fantasies and dreams. The caesarean temptation is part of the vicious circle that also includes a lack of interest in birth physiology.

6 TOWARDS A SUPER-BRAINY HOMO SAPIENS?

Should we present the age of the safe caesarean as a probable landmark in the evolution of brain size? Should we expect the advent of a super-brainy *Homo sapiens*?

INEXTENSIBLE LIMITS

Until recently it was commonly accepted that, for obstetrical reasons, the development of the human brain has reached its limits. At term, the smaller diameter of the baby's head (which is not exactly a sphere) is roughly the same as the larger diameter of the mother's pelvis (which is not exactly a cone). The evolutionary process adopted a combination of solutions in order to reach *the limits of what is possible*.

The first solution was to make pregnancy as short as possible, so that, in a sense, the human baby is born prematurely. It is as if there is a 'primal period'[1] that includes a phase of 'internal gestation' followed by a phase of 'external gestation' in a social milieu. The comparative immaturity of the human newborn baby cannot be dissociated from the development of strong social groups. I have suggested that an early birth might have multiple advantages in terms of brain development: the extrauterine world can provide a much greater variety of complex personalized sensory stimulation than the prenatal environment.[2] We have realized recently that the pregnant mother can, to a certain extent, adapt the size of the foetus to her own size by modulating the blood flow and the availability of nutrients to the foetus. That is why small surrogate mothers carrying donor embryos from much larger genetic parents give birth to smaller babies than might have been anticipated.

From a mechanical point of view, the baby's head must be as flexed as possible, so that the smaller diameter is presenting itself before spiralling down to get out of the maternal pelvis. The birth of humans is a complex asymmetrical phenomenon, the maternal pelvis being widest transversally at the entrance and widest longitudinally at the exit. A process of 'moulding' can slightly reshape the baby's skull if necessary.

When mentioning the mechanical particularities of human birth, one cannot help referring to and comparing ourselves with our close relatives the chimpanzees. The head of a baby chimpanzee at term occupies a significantly smaller space in the maternal pelvis, and the vulva of the mother is perfectly centred, so that the descent of the baby's head is as symmetrical and as direct as possible. It seems that since we separated from the other chimpanzees, and all along the evolution of the hominid species, there has been a conflict between moving upright on two feet and, at the same time, a tendency towards a larger and larger brain. The brain of the modern *Homo* is four times bigger than the brain of our famous ancestor Lucy. There is a conflict in our species because the pelvis adapted to the upright posture must be narrow to allow the legs to be close together under the spine, which facilitates transfer of forces from legs to spine when running. An upright posture is the prerequisite for brain development. We can carry heavy weights on our head when we are upright. Mammals walking on all fours cannot do the same. That is apparently why the process of evolution found other solutions than an enlarged female pelvis in order to make the birth of the 'big-brained ape' possible: the faster our ancestors could run, the more likely they were to survive.

There is another reason why one can claim that the development of brain size has reached its limits. When we refer to brain development, we are not precise enough. We should emphasize that it is not the whole brain that is dramatically developed in our species. It is that part of the brain called the neocortex. The neocortex can be presented as a sort of super computer that was originally at the service of the vital archaic brain structures. The point is that this 'new brain' tends to wield most power and that it can inhibit the activity of the primitive one, particularly during the birth process. However, modern women are still able to release the necessary hormones and give birth with their own resources, on condition that the activity of their powerful neocortex is dramatically reduced. From this point of view it appears once more that the development of the human brain has reached its limits. A still more developed neocortex might make the birth process impossible.

PULVERIZED LIMITS

All these apparently fixed limits to brain evolution are simply smashed with the advent of the safe caesarean. Until now babies who had too large a head to pass through the maternal pelvic opening did not survive birth and therefore could not transmit this tendency for larger brain size on to future generations. Today continued evolution of brain size is again possible.

We, as members of the species *Homo sapiens*, are to a great extent different from the other primates, particularly our close cousins the chimpanzees, in terms of fat metabolism. We are characterized by a huge capacity to transport fatty molecules and fatty particles to certain parts of the body, such as the skin and the brain. Only humans have a layer of fat attached to the skin and an ability to accumulate lipids in such places as breasts and buttocks for the females, and abdomen for the males. Modern life style is associated with a tendency to make the layer of fat beneath the skin thicker and thicker.

Humans are first and foremost characterized by a unique capacity to transport to the brain specific molecules of fatty acids that are necessary for its development. The developing brain has a real thirst for the fatty acid commonly called DHA: 50 per cent of the molecules of fatty acids that are incorporated into the developing brain are represented by DHA. This very long chain polyunsaturated molecule of the omega-3 family is preformed and abundant in seafood only. One of the keys to understanding human nature is to take into consideration the weakness of our delta-4 desaturation enzymes, knowing that DHA is a product of this reaction. In other words, *human beings, who are characterized by an enormous brain, are not very effective at making a molecule that is important to feed the nervous system.* This suggests that humans have been programmed to have this molecule included in their diet. In practice, this means to have access to seafood. It is justified to claim that the transmission of the tendency for larger brains is suddenly made possible at the age of the safe caesarean, particularly in populations where preformed DHA is an abundant component of the diet.

It is noticeable that the vision of the caesarean as a landmark in the evolution of brain size did not appear originally to an expert in evolutionary anthropology or an expert in childbirth. Jane English was born by non-labour classical caesarean in 1942. When she became an adult, around the age of 30, she started to use 'caesarean born' as a 'lens through which to look at the world and at herself'. This is how she realized that, while changes used to happen through mutation and natural selection, now they can be induced by the ingeniousness of humans. Her interest in the implications of being caesarean born was the reason for *Different Doorway*, the book she published in 1985.[3]

I was lucky enough to meet Jane English in the 1980s. Since that time I have started to understand why the history of childbirth is at a turning point, why the history of humankind is at a turning point, and even why the process of human evolution itself is at a turning point.

7   TWENTY-FIRST-CENTURY CRITERIA

TWO ANSWERS

Is Brazil a prototype for future-thinking nations? In cities such as Rio de Janeiro and São Paulo, a pro-caesarean culture is arising. Most women who help sway public opinion – actresses, famous athletes, etc. – give birth by caesarean. The same tendency is easily detectable in many other places throughout the world. In Taiwan, another world leader in caesarean rates, many people believe that choosing an auspicious time of birth has promising effects on children's fate. Are there serious reasons to reverse the current situation? *The answer is no, if* we take into account the sole scientific criteria of the twentieth century. These criteria are those that I have used until now in my comments on the advent of a safe technique. It is commonplace to evaluate the quality of midwifery and obstetrical practices by looking mostly at the number of babies alive at birth, the number of babies who are healthy at birth, the rates of maternal deaths and the rates of maternal complications. These include the risks of urinary incontinence, fecal incontinence and vaginal prolapse. Our comments on the evolution of brain size are also based on well-established criteria, since the Darwinian laws of evolution became better and better accepted and refined during the past century.

The answer is undoubtedly yes, if we introduce twenty-first-century criteria. I am referring in particular to the fast development of the most vital aspect of the current scientific revolution, which is *The Scientification of Love*.[1] Love was traditionally the realm of poets, artists, novelists and philosophers. At the dawn of the twenty-first century, it is being studied from a great variety of scientific perspectives. There are several reasons why it is easy to miss the importance of the phenomenon. One of them is that research is highly specialized and that experts who have detected small yet significant details are unaware of or unable to see the way their finding links up with other pieces of research.

Another reason why we are not ready to include *The Scientification of Love* in the framework of the main scientific advances is that this new generation of research *provides answers to questions that have never been raised.*

THREE QUESTIONS

The first example of a paradoxically new, yet simple, basic and necessary question is *'How does the capacity to love develop?'* Until now countless spiritual heroes, religious leaders, philosophers, poets, moralists and philanthropists of all kinds have promoted love and have encouraged the expression of the multiple facets of love, using a great diversity of terms, such as compassion, altruism, selflessness, charity, generosity, bounty, humanitarianism, mercy, empathy, sympathy and forgiveness. When considering the behaviour of twenty-first-century humans, we don't need long arguments to doubt the actual benefits of their wise words. It is now more urgent to wonder how the capacity to love develops, rather than constantly promoting love or raising negative traditional questions, such as 'How do we prevent violence?'

Today the scientification of love could prompt us to formulate questions in a positive way, because a combination of data provide answers and converge to give great importance to early experiences, particularly in the period surrounding birth. The first discipline that participated in the scientification of love is, historically speaking, ethology. Ethologists observe the behaviours of animals and human beings. Since the emergence of their discipline, they have traditionally had a particular interest in mother–baby attachment. Whatever the species of mammals they are studying, they always confirm that there is a short yet crucial period immediately after birth that will never be repeated. We must mention in particular the work of Harlow, because he looked at mother and baby monkeys, a species closely related to humans. Furthermore he followed up monkeys until adulthood and could establish correlations between different ways of disturbing the first contact between mother and baby after birth and different alterations in sexual and maternal behaviour in adulthood.

The concepts introduced by ethologists are now supported by research exploring the behavioural effects of the many hormones involved in childbirth and also in different facets of love. According to our current knowledge, when a woman is giving birth she has to release a complex cocktail of love hormones. The hormones released by mother and foetus during labour and delivery are not eliminated immediately, and each of them has a specific role to play during the hour following birth in the interaction between mother and newborn baby. These concepts are also supported by studies looking at the background of subjects who have expressed some form of impaired capacity to love (love of others and love of oneself). Such studies belong to a new framework which I call Primal Health Research and are collected in the Primal Health Research Data Bank.

Another example of a simple and new question is *What are*

the links between the many facets of love?' We use the same word for so many different situations. What are the links between maternal, paternal, filial, sexual, romantic, platonic, spiritual, brotherly love, not to mention love of country, love of inanimate objects, and compassion and concern for Mother Earth? Once more we suddenly think of raising such a question because biological sciences suggest answers.

It appears today that, whatever the facet of love, the hormone oxytocin is involved. Until recently, this hormone released by the posterior pituitary gland was known only for its mechanical effects. These well-known mechanical effects include the contraction of the uterus for the birth of the baby and the delivery of the placenta, the contraction of special breast cells so as to make the milk ejection reflex possible, the contraction of the prostate and of the seminal vesicles during the sperm ejection reflex, and also the contraction of the uterus during the female orgasm, which tends to facilitate the transportation of the sperm towards the egg. In retrospect we understand why it took a long time to demonstrate its crucial behavioural effects; it is just because oxytocin does not reach the brain as long as it is injected intravenously. The turning point came during an experiment by Pedersen and Prange, who thought of injecting oxytocin directly into the brains of virgin rats.[2] After such an injection, if there were some pups around, the virgin rats had a tendency to bring them together and take care of them. After that it did not come as a surprise to detect in the brain of mammals molecules which are sensitive to oxytocin (brain receptors). Among rats there is an increased number of oxytocin receptors during birth in a particular brain zone usually called BNST (bed nucleus of the stria terminalis). Because the experimental destruction of this zone inhibits maternal behaviour, incidentally without disturbing birth, it appears that oxytocin receptors of that zone play an important role in maternal behaviour. There are many reasons to believe that among humans brain receptors to oxytocin also develop during labour and delivery. This is one reason among others to assume that a woman develops to a certain extent her capacity to love while giving birth.

The point is that the hormone of love is always part of a complex hormonal balance. When there is a sudden release of oxytocin, the need to love can be directed in different ways depending on which other hormones are released at the same time. That is why there are different sorts of love. When there is an associated high level of prolactin, for example, the tendency is to direct the effects of the love hormone towards babies, since prolactin is the typical motherhood hormone. This is exactly what is happening immediately after a birth in physiological conditions, at a time when the peak of oxytocin can be extremely high (if the place is warm enough, if the eye-to-eye and skin-to-skin contacts between mother and baby are not disturbed, and if the sense of smell of both of them are not distracted by aggressive odours).[3,4] In other situations there is a sudden release of oxytocin without a significant amount of prolactin. It is another facet of love. It can be love for the sexual partner. Since a peak of oxytocin can participate in a quasi-infinity of possible hormonal balances, there is also a quasi-infinity of loving situations … but oxytocin is always involved.

Let us mention a last simple and new question inspired by the current scientific context: *Why do all societies ritually disturb the first contact between mother and baby?* We cannot help asking the question that way at a time when we are learning from several disciplines that the short phase of labour between the birth of the baby and the delivery of the placenta is probably critical in the development of the capacity to love. The most universal and intriguing way to disturb the so-called third stage of labour is simply to promote the belief that colostrum is

tainted or harmful to the baby – even a substance to be
expressed and discarded.[5] Let us recall that, according to
modern biological sciences, the colostrum available immediately after birth is precious. Let us also recall the newborn baby's
ability to search for the nipple and to find it as early as the first
hour following birth.[6] Several beliefs can be combined and can
reinforce each other. For example in some ethnic groups in
Benin, West Africa, they transmit the belief that the mother
must not look into the baby's eyes during the 24 hours
following birth, so that the 'bad spirits' cannot enter the baby's
body. The first contact between mother and baby can also be
disturbed through rituals: rushing to cut the cord, bathing,
rubbing, tight swaddling, foot binding, 'smoking' the baby (the
newborn is held in the smoke above a fire), piercing the ears of
little girls, and opening the doors in cold countries are examples
of such rituals.

Today, not only are we in a position to ask such a question,
but we can also offer interpretations. One must keep in mind
that for thousands of years the basic strategy for survival of
most human groups has been to dominate nature and to
dominate other human groups. There was an evolutionary
advantage in developing the human potential for aggression
rather than the capacity to love and therefore in transmitting
such beliefs and rituals. It is significant, when comparing
different societies, that the greater the need to develop aggression and the ability to destroy life, the more intrusive the rituals
and cultural beliefs are in the period around birth.

Our interpretations must be framed in the context of the
twenty-first century. We are at a time when humanity must
invent radical new strategies for survival. Today we are in the
process of realizing the limits of traditional strategies. We must
raise new questions such as 'How do we develop this form of
love which is respect for Mother Earth?' In order to stop

destroying the planet we need a sort of unification of the planetary village. We need love more than ever before. All the beliefs and rituals which challenge the maternal protective and aggressive instinct are losing their evolutionary advantages.

The age of the safe caesarean is first and foremost the age of the scientification of love. The priorities are obvious.

8   LONG-TERM THINKING

Human beings have not been programmed for long-term thinking. For millions of years our tropical ancestors consumed the food they could find from day to day in their environment, either by collecting shellfish and small fish in shallow water, by gathering plants and fruits, or by scavenging and hunting. After the comparatively recent advent of agriculture and animal breeding, they had to increase their capacity to anticipate. They were obliged to think at least in terms of seasons. Today we have at our disposal such powerful technologies that we must suddenly learn to think in terms of decades and centuries. It is so in many fields of human activities. It is so, in particular, in the field of childbirth.

A TOOL FOR REPROGRAMMING OURSELVES

It is hard to transcend human nature. Health professionals involved in childbirth cannot easily see beyond the period surrounding birth. Anyway, before the industrialization of childbirth, there was no reason and no incitement to raise questions about the possible lifelong consequences of how we are born, since everybody was born by the vaginal route, after spontaneous induction of labour, and since mother and baby had to rely on their own ability to cope with the situation. Births were just more or less difficult. Today there are many kinds of 'births from below' and many sorts of 'births from above'. Health professionals must realize that a newborn baby has a life expectancy of about 80 years.

In order to condition ourselves to think long term, we can use the Primal Health Research Data Bank as a tool (www. birthworks.org/primalhealth). Our data bank contains hundreds of references and abstracts of studies published in authoritative medical or scientific journals. All of them are about correlations between what happened during the 'primal period' and what will happen later on in life in terms of health and behaviour. (The primal period includes foetal life, the period surrounding birth and the year following birth.) It is not easy to detect such studies because they do not fit into the current classifications. This is the main reason for the data bank.

From an overview of the bank it appears immediately that, in all fields of medicine, there have been studies detecting correlations between an adult disease and what happened when the mother was pregnant. It is even possible to conclude, through this group of studies, that our health is to a great extent shaped in the womb.[1] When reading, for example, that a man is protected against the risk of having prostate cancer if his mother has had pre-eclampsia, or when reading that those who were in the womb during an epidemic of whooping cough are at increased risk of Parkinson's disease, we start training ourselves to think long-term.

BEING CAESAREAN BORN

Surprisingly enough, the keyword 'caesarean' leads us to a small number of entries. The most significant hard data we can find in the bank via this keyword relate to being caesarean born with the *risks of having asthma* in childhood and adulthood.

Finnish researchers looked at the risks of having asthma and allergic diseases among adults aged 31 (in a population born in 1966). It appeared that those born by caesarean had a risk of having asthma multiplied by 3.23 compared with those born by the vaginal route.[2] On the other hand, the risks of having allergic diseases such as hay fever or eczema, or the risks of having an allergic tendency detected by skin tests, were not increased. The same team looked at the risks of having asthma in childhood, at age seven.[3] They found that birth complications in general, and caesarean births in particular, were risk factors. Another Finnish team linked data from the 1987 National Birth Register with data from several health registers to obtain information on asthma. This study, involving nearly 60,000 children, confirmed that the risks of having asthma in childhood were increased among those born by caesarean.[4] A Danish study also found that a caesarean birth is a risk factor for asthma, but not for allergic rhinitis,[5] while a British study confirmed that there are no increased risks for allergies following a caesarean birth.[6]

When trying to interpret such convergent findings, I cannot help thinking of the well-documented fact that respiratory problems of the newborn baby are significantly more frequent after a scheduled non-labour caesarean than after a birth by the vaginal route or a caesarean during labour. Unfortunately none of these studies found in our data bank compared labour caesareans and non-labour caesareans. Today we are in a position to understand that the foetus is supposed to participate in the initiation of labour. One of the probable ways is by giving a signal, which is the release in the amniotic fluid of a substance indicating that its lungs are mature. Furthermore it seems that hormones released by mother and baby during the birth process can give a last touch to the maturation of the lungs.[7] It is therefore easy to anticipate that babies born by non-labour caesarean are more at risk of respiratory difficulties not only immediately after birth, but also later on in life.[8] It is noticeable that a caesarean birth appears as a risk factor for asthma as a respiratory disease, but not as an allergic disease.

While a caesarean birth is not a significant risk factor for allergic diseases properly speaking (those classified as atopic, such as hay fever, allergic rhinitis and eczema), it might increase the risk of food allergy. According to a Norwegian study, caesarean born children of allergic mothers are at high risk of being allergic to eggs, fish and nuts.[9]

At a time when about a million Americans and several millions Chinese are born every year 'from above', one can wonder why the keyword 'caesarean', compared with many other keywords, does not lead us to a greater number of entries. The first obvious reason is that Primal Health Research is a new discipline that has difficulties establishing itself: scientists are human beings who have not been genetically programmed to think long-term. It is significant that all papers relating to caesarean and asthma have been published after the dawn of the twenty-first century. Another reason is that most research protocols exploring risk factors in the period surrounding birth use imprecise concepts such as 'birth complications' or 'birth optimality' (scores measuring how a person was born compared with what is considered optimal). The results of this group of studies suggest that the way we are born has lifelong consequences. They open the way to another generation of research that would meet some of the main preoccupations of those who are familiar with the concept of Primal Health Research.

In the current obstetrical context, we need answers to such urgent questions as 'What are the long-term effects of being born after labour induction?' or 'What are the long-term effects of being born by non-labour caesarean?' It seems that researchers have not realized that today a great part of humanity is already born by non-labour caesarean. The medical literature cannot yet satisfy the curiosity of those who think long-term. For example, once I stumbled on a study of children whose mothers were depressed three months after giving birth; at age eleven, these children were more likely to exhibit violent behaviours, including fighting at school and using weapons during fights. My first reaction was to wonder if there is an increased risk of postnatal depression after caesarean. Not only was it difficult to find more than a couple of studies suggesting that after an emergency caesarean section the risk of maternal depression is increased (multiplied by seven according to an Australian study),[10] but it was impossible – until now – to find a study focusing on the risks after a non-labour caesarean.

IMPAIRED CAPACITY TO LOVE

In the meantime we must draw on the conclusions of studies that have already been published. An overview of the bank leads us to notice that when researchers explore the background of people who have expressed some sort of *impaired capacity to love* – either *love of oneself or love of others* – they always detect risk factors at birth. 'Impaired capacity to love' is a convenient term to underline the links between all these conditions. It includes self-destructive behaviour. That is why I present Primal Health Research as a discipline that participates in the scientification of love. Furthermore, when researchers find risk factors in the period surrounding birth, it is always about a very important issue specific to our time – either a condition which can be defined as an impaired capacity to love or a clear-cut medical condition such as asthma.

Here are typical examples of conditions I classify in the framework of impaired capacity to love: juvenile violent criminality, suicide, drug addiction, anorexia nervosa and autism. All of them have been studied from a Primal Health Research perspective.

Autism can be taken as an example to illustrate the sort of research that has already been done, and also to call attention to the need for a new generation of studies. Autism is undoubtedly topical. It can be presented as an impaired capacity to love. My interest in autism started in 1982 when I met Niko Tinbergen, one of the founders of ethology, who shared the Nobel Prize with Konrad Lorenz and Karl Von Frisch in 1973. As an ethologist familiar with the observation of animal behaviour, he studied in particular the non-verbal behaviour of autistic children. As a field ethologist he studied the children in their home environment. Not only could he offer detailed descriptions of his observations, but at the same time he listed factors which predispose to autism or which can exaggerate the symptoms.[11]

He found such factors evident in the period surrounding birth: induction of labour, deep-forceps delivery, birth under anaesthesia, and resuscitation at birth. Interestingly, this pioneer introduced the variable 'labour induction'. When I met him he was exploring possible links between difficulty in establishing eye-to-eye contact among autistic children and the absence of eye-to-eye contact between mother and baby at birth. The work of Tinbergen (and his wife) represents the first attempt to explore autism from a Primal Health Research perspective.

It is probably because I met Niko Tinbergen that I read with special attention, in June 1991, a report by Ryoko Hattori, a psychiatrist from Kumamoto, Japan.[12] She evaluated the risks of becoming autistic according to the place of birth. She found that children born in a certain hospital were significantly more at risk of becoming autistic. In that particular hospital the routine was to induce labour a week before the expected date of birth and to use a complex mixture of sedatives, anaesthesia agents and analgesics during labour. This study could not dissociate the effects of labour induction and the effects of drugs used during labour.

The largest study ever published about the perinatal risk factors for autism is dated July 2002.[13] The researchers had at their disposal the recorded data from the Swedish National Birth Register regarding all Swedish children born during a period of 20 years (from 1974 until 1993). They also had at their disposal data regarding 408 children (321 boys and 87 girls) diagnosed as autistic after being discharged from a hospital from 1987 through to 1994 (diagnosis according to strict criteria). For each case five matched controls were selected, resulting in a control sample of 2,040 infants. The risk of autism was significantly associated with caesarean delivery, a five-minute Apgar score below 7 (in other words: baby not in good shape at birth), maternal birth outside Europe and North America, bleeding in pregnancy, daily smoking in early pregnancy, being small for gestational age, and congenital malformations. Unfortunately the authors could not dissociate scheduled caesareans and caesareans during labour. Also, the labour induction variable could not be taken into account because it did not appear in the National Birth Register until 1991, as I learnt from personal correspondence with one of the authors.

Other studies (all of them much smaller than the main Swedish one) have evaluated the rates of birth complications among autistic children by using different scores of optimality. It also appears from these studies that children with what is today called autistic spectrum disorders have higher rates of birth complications. Is there a cause and effect relationship? Once more the concept of labour induction does not appear in the protocols and results of such studies, and scheduled caesareans are not dissociated from caesareans during labour.

14,15,16,17 There is food for thought in the results of a study suggesting that the symptoms of autism appear after an unusual pattern of brain growth with a sudden change after birth. During the year following birth there is a sudden and excessive increase in brain size.[18] We must keep in mind that the perinatal period is a period of reorganization of brain development. We must also give importance to the results of studies suggesting that children with autistic disorders show alterations in their oxytocin system … in the way they release their 'hormones of love'.[19] From that point of view, the period surrounding birth can also be presented as a phase of reorganization.

FROM A CUL-DE-SAC TO AN AVENUE

These studies looking at the long-term consequences of how we are born have usually been shunned by the medical community and the media, despite their publication in authoritative medical and scientific journals, and although they explore highly topical conditions. Most of them have not been replicated, even by the original investigators, and they are rarely quoted after publication.

Because I have personally met the authors of several of these studies, I can offer some comments about this family of research. I came to the conclusion that research can be politically incorrect. Most researchers looking at how people were born have faced extreme bureaucratic difficulties. It may be that they are shaking the very foundations of our societies, insofar as the birth process has always been ritually disturbed. It may also be that very few people have developed their capacity to think long-term and are ready to perceive the importance of this developing field of research, which is a new branch of epidemiology (epidemiologists study all forms of disease, states of health and behaviour that relate to the environment and ways of life). I recently coined the term 'cul-de-sac epidemiology' when referring to these studies.[20] This term contrasts with 'circular epidemiology' which has been used to describe a common and regrettable tendency to constantly repeat the same studies, even when there is no doubt about the results.

A pessimistic analysis may inspire the simplistic conclusion that politically correct research leads to circular epidemiology and that politically incorrect research leads to cul-de-sac epidemiology. I prefer to introduce an optimistic note and stress that it is possible to break through the dead end of a cul-de-sac and open an avenue. In other words the limits of political correctness are not immutable. When more researchers have developed their capacities to think long-term we'll be in a position to welcome 'breakthrough epidemiology'.

Several rules are apparent from an overview of this new generation of research. One of them is the wait-for-puberty rule. It appears from animal experiments that often the consequences of early events – such as drugs used during labour or brain lesions at the time of birth – cannot be detected until puberty. This leads to a comparison with human health conditions (for example, schizophrenia, drug addiction, anorexia, etc.) that cannot be recognized before puberty although risk factors are found during foetal life or the perinatal period. The wait-for-puberty rule leads to caution when interpreting the results of studies with a follow-up shorter than 15 years. It also leads to anticipation that there is a *future for a new branch of medicine, specialized in the diseases of adolescents.*

The new generation of research we are expecting will try to provide answers to questions of the future. Some of the new questions will be inspired by observations and experiments among mammals whose lifespan is much shorter than ours. For example, today 90 per cent of English bulldogs are born by scheduled caesarean. In addition, the English bulldog male's lack of stamina does not allow successful mating, so that artificial insemination is needed. If there is a link between these two facts, we must at least raise questions about the possible particularities of genital sexuality of a human population born by scheduled caesarean.

A COMPLEMENTARY LESSON

While browsing the data bank in order to learn about the possible long-term consequences of being caesarean born, we learn a complementary lesson. We cannot miss a group of studies that detected the possible harmful long-term effects of all sorts of difficult births by the vaginal route. Keywords such as 'forceps', 'ventouse' (or 'vacuum'), 'cephalhaematoma' or 'resuscitation' open the way to such studies. Finally, an overview of the bank provides new reasons to disturb the birth process as little as possible, and therefore new reasons to improve our understanding of the basic needs of women in labour. We might also conclude that one of the main functions of the safe modern caesarean should be to make obsolete such a tool as the forceps, which is in addition associated with the risks of serious damages of maternal tissues. Are we moving towards a *simplified two-options basic strategy*: *either* a straightforward birth by the vaginal route, *or* a caesarean during labour, if possible before the stage of emergency?

9   TOWARDS AN UNPRECEDENTED CULTURAL DIVERSITY?

THINKING IN TERMS OF CIVILIZATION

When a woman is pregnant, her main preoccupation is usually the health and wellbeing of her own baby. After the birth, the behaviour of a mother tends to be more than ever under the control of her 'selfish genes'. For her, nothing is more important than to protect her infant and to satisfy its needs. Pregnant women and young mothers *are not in a position to think in terms of civilization*. They have other understandable vital and immediate priorities.

Doctors, on the other hand, have long been under the influence of the Hippocratic ethical principles. Traditional Hippocratic medicine only considers the point of view of individual patients. There is no mention in the Hippocratic Oath of the doctor's societal responsibilities. As for the midwife, she is traditionally in intimate communication – in communion – with the labouring woman, sharing her priorities. Finally, doctors and midwives *are also not in a position to think in terms of civilization*.

BROADENING OUR HORIZON

In spite of such deep-rooted difficulties, we must all urgently broaden our horizon. The Primal Health Research perspective and statistical language both encourage us to ignore to a certain extent individuals and particular cases, by introducing the concepts of 'tendency', 'risk factors' and 'statistical significance'. In order to realize the gap between humans and other mammals and to raise the right questions, I suggest that we first refer to what we know about the effects of a caesarean among mammals in general.

A caesarean birth implies a general or a regional anaesthesia. The maternal behaviour can be dramatically disturbed just by the anaesthesia. Almost a century ago, in South Africa, Eugene Marais was conducting experiments to confirm his intuition as a poet that a connection exists between the pain of birth and maternal love.[1] He studied a group of 60 Kaffir bucks, knowing that there had not been a single instance of a buck mother in the herd rejecting her young in the previous 15 years. He proceeded to give the birthing females a few puffs of chloroform and ether, and noticed that the mothers refused to accept their newborn lambs afterwards. In the 1980s, Krehbiel and Poindron studied the effects of epidural anaesthesia among ewes giving birth.[2] The results of this study are easily summarized: when a ewe gives birth with an epidural anaesthesia, she doesn't take care of her lamb.

Today cesarean sections are common in veterinary medicine, particularly among dogs. This is possible as long as human beings compensate for frequently inadequate maternal behaviour, assist the process of nursing and provide, if necessary, commercial canine milk replacers. The effects of a caesarean on the maternal behaviour of primates are well-documented, because several species of monkeys are used as laboratory animals. This is the case of the crab-eating macaques and the rhesus monkeys.[3] In these species the mothers do not take care of their babies after a caesarean; laboratory personnel must spread vaginal secretions on the baby's body in order to try to induce the mother's interest for her newborn.

We don't need to multiply the examples of animal experiments and observations by veterinarians and primate-using scientists to convince anyone that a caesarean – or just the anaesthesia that is necessary for the operation – can dramatically alter the maternal behaviour of mammals in general.

In this regard humans are special. Millions of women all over the world have taken care of their baby after a caesarean birth or simply an epidural birth or a 'twilight sleep birth'.

We know why the behaviour of humans is more complex and more difficult to interpret than the behaviour of other mammals, including primates. Human beings have developed sophisticated ways to communicate. They speak. They create cultures. Their behaviour is influenced less directly by their hormonal balance and more directly by the cultural milieu. When a woman knows that she is expecting a baby, she can anticipate displaying some maternal behaviour. This does not mean that we cannot learn from non-human mammals. The spectacular and immediate behavioural responses of animals indicate the questions we should raise about ourselves.

Where human beings are concerned, the questions must include terms such as 'civilization' or 'culture'. If other mammals do not take care of their babies after a caesarean, we must first wonder: *What is the future of a civilization born by caesarean?*

TOWARDS DIFFERENT 'NATIVE' CULTURES?

For obvious reasons we cannot yet provide precise answers to such a question. The safe caesarean as a consumer good is too recent in the history of humankind. There is no cultural model.

In the meantime, we can study the main characteristics of different cultures in relation to how babies are born by exploring specialized databases. It is noticeable that the greater the need a society has to develop aggression and the ability to destroy life, the more intrusive the rituals and cultural beliefs are in the period around birth. Let us combine this data with what we learn from Primal Health Research about the root of different sorts of impaired capacity to love, and also from other disciplines that participate in the scientification of love. It is becoming possible today to anticipate what kind of effects the widespread use of the caesarean may have on the evolution of the cultural milieux. These effects should be mostly in terms of sociability, capacity to love others, and also capacity to love oneself. Self-esteem and self-image are well-documented components of the capacity to love oneself.

There are such differences in the rates of caesareans between countries that we should not have to wait many decades before being able to compare tendencies in the evolution of cultural milieux. How will the Dutch vaginally born culture evolve compared with the Brazilian caesarean born culture? How will the Japanese culture evolve compared with the Taiwanese or South Korean? Our genetically limited capacity to think long-term can explain why there is not already an army of experts in human sciences raising such questions and looking at detectable tendencies.

While waiting for a new awareness that will reach and influence the scientific community, let us listen again to Jane English, who was non-labour caesarean born in 1942, and who is using caesarean born as a lens to look at the world. Although she is scientifically minded, having a doctorate in sub-atomic physics, her approach did not lead her to conduct what we are inclined to call 'scientific studies'. After self-exploration and after collecting anecdotal material, she thinks of caesarean birth

(particularly non-labour caesarean birth) as creating a different
native culture, the word native being used in the literal sense of
having to do with birth. One of her conclusions is that
non-labour caesarean birth creates a different view of space and
time, with different personal boundaries.[4] She distances herself
from the widespread tendency to use the concept of cause and
effect relationship in one way only. She dares to claim that not
only is caesarean birth a cause of personality traits, it is also
itself an effect of them. Her unwonted viewpoint inspires
questions such as 'Why 10 per cent caesarean rates in Amsterdam and 80 per cent in São Paulo?'

Travellers should already be aware of the huge cultural gap
between Amsterdam and São Paulo, for example. We can walk
at night in the streets of Amsterdam. It would be suicidal to do
so in São Paulo. Any conclusion would be premature.

The concept of native culture might be instrumental for
interpreting the fast recent evolution of certain cultural milieux.
Let us consider, for example, the emergence of the drug culture
in the US, around 1970. It is noticeable that this particular
generation of Americans was born at the age of 'twilight sleep
deliveries' (twilight sleep implies the use, during labour, of
morphine associated with other drugs). The link between these
two facts becomes highly plausible when taking into account a
series of Swedish studies (by Bertil Jacobson and Karin Nyberg)
included in the Primal Health Research data bank. According to
these studies, when a woman in labour has used certain
painkillers (particularly morphine-like substances) her child is,
statistically speaking, more at risk of becoming drug addicted.

Let us consider, as another example, the 10–20 per cent
annual increase in volume during the past ten years of *plastic
surgery procedures in Brazil*. Brazil now ranks second behind
the US in terms of number of cosmetic plastic surgery procedures. This prompted Mara Cristina Souza de Lucia, chief

psychologist of Clinicas Hospital at the University of São Paulo, to evaluate self-image among 346 normal-weight men and women.[5] Her team of researchers found that 50 per cent were unsatisfied with their body and 67 per cent of women and 28 per cent of men would like to have plastic surgery. Lucia commented: 'Some of them go from doctor to doctor ... but they are never satisfied with their looks.' Is this an expression of a widespread impaired capacity to love oneself?

Today, for the first time in the history of humankind, there are many ways to be born. Within the only framework of caesarean births, we must distinguish non-labour C-sections from in-labour C-sections and emergency C-sections. Whatever the final route, we must also distinguish induced labour from spontaneous labour. Among the vaginal births, some are drugless while many others combine in different ways epidural anaesthesia and a drip of synthetic oxytocin ...

Is humanity evolving towards an unprecedented diversity of 'native cultures'?

10 ENTERING THE WORLD OF MICROBES

TWO DOORWAYS TOWARDS THE WORLD OF MICROBES

To be born is also to enter the world of microbes. At the very time when the baby is getting out of the mother's body, its digestive tract and all its mucous membranes are germ-free. Some hours later, there will be billions of germs in its nose, in its mouth and in its gut. The main question is *which germs will be the first to colonize the baby's body*?

This question is important because, for the newborn baby, certain germs are already familiar and friendly, while others are unfamiliar and potentially dangerous. The reason is that the human placenta is very active at transferring maternal antibodies commonly called IgG. Since the newborn baby has the same levels of such antibodies as its mother, this implies that the microbes that are familiar to the mother are also familiar to the germ-free newborn baby. Among humans this transfer of antibodies is particularly intense from 38 weeks onward.[1] It is worth noticing that high levels of such antibodies at birth (often higher than the maternal levels) is a specifically human trait. These levels are much lower at birth among primitive primates such as squirrel monkeys.[2]

A well-known concept used by bacteriologists is another reason to give great importance to the nature of the first germs that will colonize the baby's body. 'The race for the surface' means that the winners of the race to reach a germ-free territory will likely be the rulers of the territory. This concept can have practical implications. During epidemics in nurseries it was found that the colonization of babies with virulent staphylococci could be prevented by early voluntary contamination (nasal or umbilical) with a strain of staphylococcus selected because of its very low virulence and its great susceptibility to penicillin.[3]

It is therefore clear that, from a bacteriological point of view, a newborn baby urgently needs to be in contact with only one person – her mother. It is also clear that, *from a bacteriological point of view, there is an inherent and fundamental difference between a vaginal birth and a caesarean birth*. The human mammal had been programmed to enter the world via an orifice situated close to the maternal anus. This is a sort of guarantee that the newborn baby – particularly her digestive tract – will be immediately contaminated by a great variety of friendly germs carried by her mother. The baby born by caesarean enters the world of microbes in a radically different way. She is born in the sterile environment of an operating room. She is more likely first to meet the microbes that are in the air of a high-tech hospital and those that are transferred by the nursing staff. She is less likely to find the breast and to consume the early colostrum, which contains specific antibodies (IgA) and other anti-infectious substances. For all these reasons the gut flora of a caesarean born is different from what it would be after a birth in physiological conditions. A delayed or aberrant colonization of the newborn intestine has been offered as an explanation for the increased risk of food allergy of caesarean born children whose mothers were allergic.[4]

GUT FLORA AND HEALTH

The way human beings establish their gut flora during the hours following birth is a serious issue. First, a healthy gut flora is a powerful barrier against a great number of pathogenic bacteria. It is vital for making vitamins and breaking down toxins. Furthermore, it plays an important role in the development and the maturation of the immune system. Any question about the development of health leads us to consider how the gut flora is established when the baby enters the world of microbes. There are many sorts of lymphocytes, a group of cells with immune action. Good health implies a certain balance between those called TH1 and those called TH2. At birth, the TH2 response is preponderant. A healthy gut flora tends to rapidly deviate the immune system towards the other direction. If this deviation does not occur at the right time there is a theoretical increased risk of certain forms of allergy afterwards. It is noticeable that a caesarean appears as a risk factor for asthma (www.birthworks.org/primalhealth). It is also noticeable that a BCG – the vaccine for protection against tuberculosis (TB) – at birth seems to moderate the risk of asthma in childhood.[5] This practice can be seen as a way of bringing a family of bacteria that are missing in a hospital environment and that deviate the immune system towards TH1. This effect might be a way to compensate the consequences of 'birth from above', and of childbirth in a high-tech environment in general. This effect has nothing to do with the prevention of TB.

It is not yet well understood that the enormous gut flora (weighing up to 2 kg) is an aspect of the personality of a human being. Today there is a great interest in manipulating this microflora with probiotic products provided by yoghurts, drinks and supplements.[6] In fact it is unlikely that the bacteria contained in probiotic products could bring about permanent changes to a healthy microflora that has been established to a great extent immediately after birth, and that is highly influenced by the method of infant feeding. This leads to another question: is it easy to breastfeed after a caesarean delivery?

11 ENTERING THE WORLD OF ODOURS

STARTING FROM ANECDOTES

In 1977, in Rome, at a congress of Psychosomatic Obstetrics and Gynaecology, I spoke about the various environmental conditions so that the baby can find the breast during the hour following birth.[1] In the scientific context of that time I could only refer to personal observations and anecdotes. I had noticed that newborn babies do not find the nipple easily when the birthing room has been recently cleaned and when aggressive odours have not yet completely disappeared. Furthermore, I had been intrigued by several anecdotes suggesting that the sense of smell of a woman who is giving birth or who has just given birth is highly sensitive.

Once a labouring woman was adamant that there was an odour of cigarette smoke in the birthing room. It was politely explained to her why this was impossible. However, we realized afterwards that a worker had spent some minutes in the room the day before, just to replace a bulb: he had the breath of a smoker. Such anecdotes lead to the practical consideration of creating a favourable olfactive climate in the birthing room and to the conclusion that 'all strong smells characteristic of a hospital environment must be eliminated, and the number of people in the room reduced to as few as possible'. I was already in a position to assume that the sense of smell probably is 'one of the best conductors towards the nipple, and is perhaps one of the newborn's first ways of identifying the mother'.

There were many reasons why my paper was deemed strange. In 1977, most obstetricians, paediatricians, midwives, nurses and lay people had never heard of a newborn baby finding the nipple during the hour following birth. They had never seen a newborn baby staying continuously in the arms of an ecstatic mother, in a quasi-sacred atmosphere. It had always been routine to 'take care' of the baby before showing her to the mother. At that time we were still under the influence of the long-held belief that odours are of little importance for human behaviour. We were still in the grip of all the cross-cultural rituals and beliefs whose effects are to separate mother and baby immediately after birth.

IN THE CURRENT SCIENTIFIC CONTEXT

In the current scientific context, we can easily explain that to be born is also to enter the world of odours. At the very time when the baby is entering the atmosphere and breathing starts, the mucous membranes of its nose are suddenly exposed, for the first time, to volatile compounds. Before birth the sensitive receptors of the nose have already been stimulated by a great variety of substances in the amniotic fluid and by blood-borne substances. But this was not smelling. The sense of smell is related to airborne compounds.

Plugs blocking the nostril of the foetus resolve in the middle of intrauterine life. This marks the beginning of the fast development of what will be the sense of smell, which appears as one of the most primitive sensory functions.

Clear responses to strong odourants have been reported in premature babies born more than two months before the due date.[2] The organization of the olfactory system is now studied in depth.

We have learnt recently that no less than 1–2 per cent of our genes seem to be allocated to the production of a rich array of specific receptors that bind odorous molecules.[3] Their activation mediates the sense of smell. It also mediates endocrine responses. It appears in particular that there are strong connections between the olfactory system (sense of smell) and the release of the love hormone oxytocin.[4] There are also strong connections between the olfactory system and a brain centre involved in the release of noradrenaline, a hormone of the adrenaline family. This hormone facilitates olfactory learning.[5,6] If we recall that during the first hour following birth the levels of noradrenaline in the baby's blood are increased 20–30-fold compared to later life, we are in a position to understand how newborn babies are physiologically prepared to learn to recognize the olfactory signature of their mother.

These theoretical considerations suggest that the role of the sense of smell for human behaviour has been traditionally ignored, particularly in the period surrounding birth.

There has recently been an explosion in experimental studies confirming the newborn's capacity to make olfactory discrimination. These studies also indicate that *naturally occurring odours* play an important role in the behaviour of the baby. Recent data have demonstrated the specific interest of the newborn baby in the odours coming from the amniotic fluid.[7,8,9,10] The mother, whose sense of smell is so acute in the period surrounding birth, also seems to be particularly sensitive to the odour of the amniotic fluid. Immediately after birth, I heard women still 'on another planet' looking in their baby's eyes and saying: 'What a sweet smell!' There have been also studies confirming the interest of the baby in the smell of the nipple,[11] and the armpit.[12]

If naturally occurring odours significantly influence the interaction between mother and newborn baby, we must acknowledge that there is a fundamental and irreducible difference between a birth 'from above' in an operating room and a non-medicated birth in a less clinical environment. We have many reasons to wonder whether it is easy to breastfeed after a caesarean delivery. We have many reasons to raise unwonted questions. My French origins urge me to ask myself: 'What is the future of gastronomy in a caesarean-born culture?'

12 NURSING THE
CAESAREAN BORN

Women have been programmed to give birth thanks to the release of a flow of hormones. The same hormones are involved in lactation. The strong connections between the birth process and the initiation of lactation make inevitable a series of questions about nursing the caesarean born.

LACTATION STARTS BEFORE THE BABY IS BORN

There are many examples of easy-to-explain connections between the physiology of birth and the physiology of lactation.

Mammals in general and women in particular control the pain of labour by releasing morphine-like substances called endorphins.[1,2] It has been demonstrated that these endorphins stimulate the secretion of prolactin, the key hormone of lactation.[3] It is therefore possible today to interpret a chain of events which starts with the physiological pain of labour and leads to the release of a hormone considered necessary for the *secretion* of milk.

The same hormone – oxytocin – is necessary for the contraction of the uterus during labour, and also for the contraction of the breast during the milk *ejection* reflex, when the baby is sucking. It is debatable whether women who have had no labour can release oxytocin as effectively as those who gave birth in physiological conditions. A Swedish study provides answers to this question by taking into account the fact that oxytocin must be released through frequent pulsations in order to be effective. This study found that two days after birth, when the baby is at the breast, women who gave birth vaginally released oxytocin in a very pulsatile – and therefore effective – way, compared with women who gave birth by emergency caesarean section.[4] Furthermore, according to this study, there is a correlation between the way oxytocin is released two days after birth and the duration of exclusive breastfeeding. In other words, the duration of breastfeeding seems to depend on how the baby was born. The same Swedish team found that the caesarean women lacked a significant rise in prolactin levels at 20–30 minutes after the onset of breastfeeding.

Let us comment also on the findings of an Italian study, according to which the amount of endorphins in the milk of the first days is much higher among mothers who gave birth vaginally compared with mothers who underwent caesarean section.[5] It is probable that one of the effects of morphine-like substances is to induce a sort of addiction to mother's milk. One can anticipate that the more addicted to the breast the newborn baby becomes, the longer and easier the breastfeeding.

In general it is easy to explain that the first time when the human neonate is able to find the breast,[6] the behaviour of mother and baby is influenced by the numerous hormones they released during labour and delivery.[7] These different hormones released by mother and baby during the birth process are still present or rebound during the hour following birth, and all of them play a specific role in the interaction between mother and baby and therefore the initiation of lactation. There is an accumulation of data confirming that, in general, a caesarean born baby (particularly a baby born after a non-labour caesarean) is physiologically different from a baby born by the vaginal route. The lungs and heart do not work in the same way.[8] The glucose levels tend to be lower.[9] Babies born by elective caesarean tend to have a lower body temperature during the first 90 minutes following birth, compared with babies born by the vaginal route or by caesarean during labour.[10]

LOOKING FOR CONFIRMATION

These theoretical considerations lead me to suspect that a caesarean delivery, particularly a scheduled caesarean, should make breastfeeding more difficult and also shorter in duration. This is also confirmed by countless anecdotes and by word of mouth. But we cannot rely on anecdotes. Any thesis can be supported by well-selected anecdotes. There are women who can breastfeed without any difficulty for several years after a scheduled caesarean, while others have major breastfeeding complications after a non-medicated vaginal birth. On the other hand, statistical studies are difficult to interpret, because they cannot be randomized. This means that the first step cannot be to draw lots in order to divide a population in two groups. For example, one cannot ask one thousand women, at random, to give birth by caesarean, while others, also at random, will be supposed to give birth by the vaginal route. The quality and the duration of breastfeeding should also be influenced by the method of anaesthesia. A Danish study compared 28 women who had a caesarean with an epidural and 28 women who had a caesarean with general anaesthesia. Women who had an epidural breastfed longer (at six months: 71 per cent versus 39 per cent).[11]

Once more we can learn from Brazil. We presented Brazil as a country where the rates of caesareans are skyrocketing and where the pro-caesarean mentality has become pervasive. It is also a country where breastfeeding promotion has been institutionalized. This mere correlation provides food for thought. The PNIAM (Programa Nacional o Incentivo ao Aleitamento Materno) was established in 1981 and included in the 1988 Brazilian constitution. This programme was noted for its intensity, extent, and innovation. Each state organized training for all categories of health professionals and also for traditional healers and others in the alternative health sector. High-profile mass media campaigns featured national celebrities, and legislation was passed on issues such as the advertising of breast milk, substitutes and increased maternity leave. Brazil has also been an active participant in the Baby Friendly Hospital Initiative, and in 1998 had achieved 103 accredited hospitals. This combination of high rates of caesarean and intense breastfeeding promotion stimulates our curiosity about how Brazilian babies are nursed.

Almeida and Couto conducted an interesting survey about lactation among Brazilian women health professionals whose mission is to recommend exclusive breastfeeding for six months.[12] When these experts in lactation had their own babies the average duration of exclusive breastfeeding was a mere 98 days! All these women had a guaranteed 120-day maternity leave. A 'detail' was mentioned in the report of this study: among university-level health professionals, *85.7 per cent* had had *C-sections*, as compared with *66.7 per cent* among technical health professionals. In general, official brazilian statistics look at the prevalence of breastfeeding rather than at the duration of exclusive breastfeeding.[13] An inquiry about weaning practices in northeast Brazil (where 99 per cent of women breastfeed when leaving hospital) revealed that the median age for starting 'other' milk was 24 days.[14] Such data support what we understand from the physiological perspective and tend to confirm that prolonged exclusive breastfeeding is not easy in a country where most babies are 'born from above'.

Let us contrast the lesson from Brazil with a lesson from Jeddah, Saudi Arabia, a place where 40 per cent babies are still breastfed at twelve months, and where the rates of caesareans are only 13 per cent. A caesarean is the main factor associated with early interruption of breastfeeding.[15] Let us mention also that Scandinavian countries combine high rates of breastfeeding and moderate rates of caesareans.

At a time when a great proportion of the world population is born by caesarean, there is an urgent need for in-depth research exploring the links between birth and lactation. Today the priority is not to constantly repeat that 'Breast is Best'. It is to wonder how the capacity to breastfeed develops.

FROM A PRACTICAL POINT OF VIEW

Breastfeeding after a caesarean is new. Most women who had a caesarean before 1980 did not breastfeed. According to a British evaluation, a mere 2 per cent of caesarean mothers breastfed their baby in 1975.[16] This was a time when 'humanized' milk formulas were developing, breastfeeding was devalued, caesareans were usually performed under general anaesthesia and their rates were still comparatively low. In such a context there was no incitement to challenge the widespread belief that women cannot breastfeed after giving birth via the abdominal route.

Today, in many countries, most mothers breastfeed after a caesarean. The initiation of lactation cannot be the same as after a birth in physiological conditions. After a non-medicated birth by the vaginal route, it is usually better to guide the beginning of breastfeeding as little as possible and to rely on continuous mother–baby contact in an atmosphere of complete privacy. After a caesarean, for obvious reasons, mother and baby need help.

In a situation of emergency, a general anaesthetic may be the easiest to administer, but it makes the mother unconscious for the birth and drowsy for some time after. However, I know from experience that many babies can actively suck the nipple about two hours after a caesarean with a short and light general anaesthesia. Today, in the usual case of an epidural or spinal anaesthesia, some women can suckle their babies while still on the operating table. In fact, if I take into account both my own experience and other accounts I've heard, it seems more important, where the initiation of lactation is concerned, to contrast caesarean during labour and scheduled caesarean, rather than focusing on the kind of anaesthesia that has been used. *Non-labour caesareans* seem to be associated with *more breastfeeding difficulties*. It is easy to offer an interpretation: when the time of birth has been planned, mother and baby have not been given the opportunity to release the hormones involved in both childbirth and lactation. Surprisingly, I could find only one study addressing this issue. This study from Ankara, Turkey, compared the starting time of lactation and the amount of milk produced within 24 hours among several groups of caesarean births.[17] The beginning of lactation was found to occur earlier and the amount of milk produced to be higher among women whose second caesarean was performed during labour, compared with women whose second caesarean was scheduled.

During the first days, most women need help, at least until the time when they can pass their intestinal gas. This is really the turning point in terms of comfort and well-being, as after any abdominal operation. Women need someone to pass the baby to them, to arrange the pillows and to position the baby for feeds. During the very first days, feeding while lying down often appears as the best position. The nurse who brings the baby can help the mother to be comfortable and to roll over to feed from the other breast. After the first days, women become more audacious and experiment with nursing positions that are most comfortable for them. Probably because the perineum is not sore after a caesarean, many women are comfortable sitting in a low chair or even cross-legged, in the tailor fashion (this does not imply that the perineum is always sore after a vaginal birth).

Because caesarean mothers and babies need to be more persevering and determined than others, they should be encouraged to share their problems and participate in support groups when this is locally possible.

13 A THOUSAND AND ONE REASONS TO BE OFFERED A CAESAREAN

Many of the women who will have a baby in the near future will be offered a caesarean. It would take volumes to analyse all the possible situations. There are several ways to classify the reasons for 'birth from above'. We'll contrast absolute indications and debatable indications.

ABSOLUTE INDICATIONS

Mothers-to-be need to be well aware of some definite and undisputable indications, even though they represent a tiny proportion of all births.

Cord prolapse belongs to this group. Occasionally, when the bag of water ruptures – artificially or spontaneously – the cord slips through the cervix into the vagina and may appear at the vulva. It becomes vulnerable to compression and the supply of blood to the baby can be cut off. This is an indisputable indication for caesarean … except if the labour is so advanced that the baby is born right away. In the case of a baby head-first at term, cord prolapse is exceptionally rare if the bag of water has not been ruptured artificially. It is more common in premature labour or if a foot presents first. During the minutes preceding the emergency caesarean, an all-fours posture can reduce pressure on the cord.

In the case of a *real placenta praevia* the afterbirth is covering the cervix so that the baby's exit is blocked. The most typical signs are bright red, painless bleeding, usually at night in late pregnancy. An ultrasound scan confirms the position of the placenta. A real placenta praevia is a diagnosis of late pregnancy. It is an absolute indication for caesarean. When a mid-pregnancy scan detects a low insertion, it is highly probable that the placenta will move upwards to a more normal position during the following weeks. The term 'placenta praevia' should not be used in mid-pregnancy.

A *placenta abruption* can occur before or during labour. It means that all of the placenta, or a great part of it, separates from the uterine wall before the baby is born. In the typical and spectacular form, there is a sudden and terrible abdominal pain. This pain is continuous, without any remission. It is some-times, but not always, accompanied by bleeding. The mother may be in a state of shock. It is often not known why placenta abruption occurs, while in some cases the cause seems obvious: for example, a trauma (such as a road accident or the effect of domestic violence) or the disease pre-eclampsia. In this spec-tacular form, when the bleeding is more or less concealed, without avenue of escape, the usual emergency treatment is blood transfusion and very fast caesarean while the baby is still alive. In fact there are many mild forms which can be related to the separated edge of the placenta, usually with painless haemorrhage. Today these mild forms may be recognized by ultrasound scanning. In general, if placenta abruption is the reason why the doctor suggests a caesarean section, it is better not to dispute the indication. Premature separation of the placenta remains one of the main causes of intrauterine death.

A *brow presentation* means that the head of the baby is midway between full flexion (the usual vertex presentation) and complete extension (the face presentation). Diagnosis of brow presentation can occasionally be suspected by abdominal palpation: a prominence (the occiput) is encountered along the foetal back. It is usually diagnosed in advanced labour by vaginal examination: the orbital ridge, eyes and even nose can be reached with a finger. In the case of a brow presentation the largest diameter of the foetal head (from occiput to chin) is the presenting portion. A persistent brow presentation in advanced labour is an absolute indication for caesarean.

A *transverse lie* is the same as a *shoulder presentation*. It means that the baby is lying horizontally, neither head-down, nor bottom-down. In the case of a woman who is not expecting her first baby, the foetus is more likely to move into a longitudinal position towards the end of pregnancy or at the very beginning of labour. If not, there is no way that a baby in such a position can be born vaginally. It is another absolute indication for caesarean. The technique of caesarean must often be modified in the case of a transverse lie, because the low segment of the uterus does not develop properly if neither the head nor the bottom are the presenting part. The trick I have used several times is to expand the transverse uterine incision into an inverted T, thanks to a short branch running up vertically on the midline.

Cardiac arrest occurs about once in every 30,000 late pregnancies. If basic life support is not immediately effective, the timing of caesarean and the speed with which surgical delivery is carried out is critical in determining the outcome for mother and baby. Most of the children and mothers who survive emergency caesarean are delivered within five minutes of maternal cardiac arrest.[1]

DEBATABLE INDICATIONS

While absolute indications are extremely rare, the most usual reasons for having a caesarean are highly influenced by a great diversity of factors such as the personality, age and experience of the midwife and the doctor; the country where the birth occurs; the local hospital protocols and fashions; the personality, the standard of living, the family background and the circle of friends of the mother-to-be; the latest studies published in authoritative medical journals; the latest study reported by the media; and the information provided by a popular website, etc. That is why the rates of caesareans vary enormously from obstetrician to obstetrician, from hospital to hospital and from country to country.

Having a uterine scar (usually a *previous caesarean*) is a significant example of relative and debatable indication, with rising and falling rates according to the phase of the history of childbirth. Today the focus is shifting towards the risks of unexplained stillbirth, although the absolute risks are very small.[2] Having a previous caesarean is such a common situation and such a topical issue that we'll look at it separately.

'Failure to progress' is a frequent recorded reason for a first caesarean section. Most cases of failure to progress are related to the current widespread misconceptions of birth physiology. It will take decades to rediscover that human beings are mammals and that the basic need of mammals giving birth is privacy. It will take decades to realize that a midwife was originally a mother-figure, that is to say the kind of person with whom one feels secure without feeling observed and judged. In the current context it would be dangerous to establish as a primary objective a reduction in the rate of caesareans. The immediate effect would be to multiply risky interventions by the vaginal route

and to increase the number of babies who need to be transferred into paediatrics. Meanwhile we must accept that most caesareans are necessary in the age of industrialized childbirth and that failure to progress is the most frequent indication.

Cephalopelvic disproportion (commonly called CPD) simply means that the baby's head is too large to fit through the mother's pelvis. It is a vague concept because the fit between a baby and a mother's pelvis depends to a great extent on the exact position of the head and how the head is moulding during labour. In the case of a caesarean decided during labour, it is difficult to dissociate CPD and failure to progress because afterwards, in similar circumstances, one or the other of the two reasons may be electively given to the mother.

Foetal distress is also a vague concept, since not all health professionals use the same criteria to make this diagnosis. Foetal distress during labour is often related to failure to progress. This is why it is artificial to dissociate these two issues. Today labour induction is a frequent risk factor for what is finally recorded as failure to progress, cephalopelvic disproportion or foetal distress.

Fibroids and *ovarian cysts* are not absolute indications, except if they are large and low, blocking the passage of the baby down the birth canal.

A *previous anal sphincter rupture* is also a debatable indication for caesarean section. According to an American study, only two caesareans are needed to prevent one case of anal incontinence among women who had previously suffered a sphincter rupture.[3]

Breech presentation offers the most typical example of the impact that one published study can have overnight all over the world. Without being simplistic, we can claim that the turning point in the history of breech birth came on 21 October, 2000. On that day, the *Lancet* – one of the most prestigious medical journals in the world – published a large trial involving 121 hospitals in 26 countries.[4] This study had a high scientific value because it was randomized, which means that, after drawing lots, the researchers divided a population of pregnant women into two groups. This is how they could compare a policy of planned caesarean section with a policy of planned vaginal birth. They studied only frank and complete breech presentations at term. Frank breech means buttocks first, with hips flexed and knees extended, so that the legs are like splints along the baby's trunk. Complete breech means that hips and knees are flexed, but the feet are not below the baby's buttocks. Footling presentations, when one or two feet are below the buttocks, were excluded from this trial.

This is how the authors of this study summarized their conclusions: 'Planned caesarean section is better than planned vaginal birth for the term foetus in the breech presentation; serious maternal complications are similar between the groups.'

As a result of this study it is difficult today to find an obstetrician who would accept the responsibility of a breech birth by the vaginal route. The quasi-standard strategy is to try to turn the baby three to four weeks before the due date. If it does not work, a scheduled caesarean is advised.

If we take into account the widespread misconceptions regarding birth physiology, we must accept that, today, it is usually better to give birth by caesarean to a breech baby rather than to try the vaginal route in the presence of apprehensive practitioners. This will remain true as long as the basic needs of labouring women, particularly the need for privacy, have not been rediscovered. There are women who accept the principle of a caesarean birth but, intuitively or in a rational way, they feel that it would be more beneficial for the baby to wait for the beginning of labour. This point of view is shared by many paediatricians who emphasize that the risks of respiratory difficulties are lower after in-labour caesarean. We must keep in mind that the alleged advantage of hospital birth is the possibility of performing an operation at any time, day or night. It is often claimed that an emergency caesarean is associated with more maternal complications than a scheduled caesarean. But *in-labour caesarean* should not be confused with *emergency caesarean*.

Today we must also think of women who, in spite of all opposition, want to avoid a caesarean section and try the vaginal route.[5] I find it useful to transmit some simple rules that I gradually adopted as a result of attending about 300 breech births by the vaginal route (including two home births):

- The best possible environment is usually a place with no one present except an experienced, motherly, silent and low-profile midwife who is not scared by a breech birth.

- The first stage of labour is a trial. If it is straightforward, easy and fast, the vaginal route is possible. If the first stage is long and difficult, a caesarean should be decided upon without any delay, before the point of no return has been reached.

- Because the first stage is a trial, it is important not to make it artificially too easy, either with drugs or even with water immersion.

- After the point of no return, privacy remains the keyword. The priority is to make the birth as easy and fast as possible. Even listening to the heartbeat is a useless and even counter-productive distraction. Creating the conditions for a powerful foetus ejection reflex should be the main objective.[6]

- It is permissible to be more audacious with a frank breech than with the other varieties of breech presentation.

The strategies adopted for breech births have significant effects on overall caesarean rates, since breech presentations at term represent about 3 per cent of all births.

There are more and more caesareans for *twin births*. One of the reasons for this new tendency is that one of the babies is breech in about 40 per cent of twin births, while both present breech about 8 per cent of the time.[7] There is even an increased tendency to schedule a caesarean when one of the babies is much bigger than the other, a situation that is considered potentially dangerous for the smaller baby, particularly in same-sex twin pregnancies. The concept of scheduled caesarean for twins may catch unawares those who keep in mind that the main preoccupation is the risk of prematurity. There are also occasional reasons to rescue a second twin by caesarean after the first one was born vaginally. The birth of the second twin is usually considered more risky than the birth of the first one. One of the reasons why the birth of the second one may be more difficult is the usual and irrational agitation in the birthing room as soon as the first twin is born, at the very time when it would be so important to maintain a quasi-sacred atmosphere, at least until the second birth and the delivery of the placenta. Once more the current tendencies are related to the widespread lack of understanding of the function of privacy.

Today *triplets* are almost always born by caesarean, even if this policy has been occasionally questioned and if there are reported anecdotes of spontaneous deliveries … including triplets born at home after a previous caesarean![8]

There is also an increasing trend of caesarean deliveries in *HIV-infected women*. The objective is to reduce the risks of transmission of the virus from mother to baby. This indication is another example of how the practices can change overnight in the age of evidence-based medicine. From 1994 to 1998, the caesarean rates among HIV-infected women in the US were stable at around 20 per cent. In 1998, published studies found that the risks were significantly reduced by avoiding the vaginal route. After that, between 1998 and 2000, the rates were around 50 per cent.[9] They probably still increase with the advent of an adapted technique protecting the baby from any contact with maternal blood. The *herpes virus* could also be transferred to the baby during a vaginal delivery. More often than not, the herpes is recurrent. This means that the mother had several episodes before being pregnant. In this case the risks of transmission are almost non-existent, because the mother has had the time to develop the kinds of antibodies that cross the placenta (IgG) and therefore protect the baby. The risks are more serious in the unusual case of a first episode during the pregnancy; in such a situation the mother has only developed the sort of antibodies, called IgM, that do not cross the placenta. Then a caesarean can reduce the risks of transmission.

And what about *vulnerable babies*, particularly those *born prematurely* and those who are 'small-for-date'? So much contradictory data has been published that any doctor can always find studies supporting their attitude. And what about the 'special' baby who is the result of years of treatment for infertility followed by a sophisticated method of medically assisted conception? And that other 'special' baby conceived just after an unexplained stillbirth?

In the future, if the basic needs of labouring women are not urgently rediscovered, and if the perineal route is more often that not presented as a risk factor for a great diversity of body damages and diseases,[10] I wonder if it will not be easier and faster to look at the remaining reasons for a vaginal birth, rather than trying to analyse the thousand and one possible indications for a caesarean.

14   ONCE A CAESAREAN
ALWAYS A CAESAREAN?

In 1916 Edwin Cragin made his historical statement in a presentation, 'Once a caesarean, always a caesarean', to the Eastern Medical Society of New York.[1] This dictum was perfectly appropriate at a time when the extremely rare caesareans were performed with a classical incision, via the direct route. The risks of a life-threatening bloody form of uterine rupture was in the region of 12 per cent.

AFTER 1950

In the 1950s, when the low-segmental incision started to gradually replace the classical one, the obstetrical edit might have been reconsidered right away, since one of the alleged advantages of the new technique was to make the uterine scar safe. However, most practitioners remained cautious and were not ready to reconsider overnight a deeply engraved dictum. The dictum had been completed by the tacit, well-accepted rule that three caesareans was the limit in the life of a woman. It is worth mentioning that at least one audacious woman has scorned this rule, since Ethel Kennedy, the wife of Robert Kennedy, gave birth to her eleven children by caesarean between 1951 and 1968.

Until 1980, only a small number of women had a vaginal birth after caesarean (VBAC). The American rate of VBAC in

1980 was only 3.4 per cent. This was before the age of what we call today evidence-based medicine. VBAC was not yet topical. Doctors were guided by word of mouth, by anecdotes and by their own belief. It became topical, particularly in the US, when the caesarean rates were climbing and when more and more women wanted to avoid a repeated section. More often than not, these mothers could not find a doctor who accepted the principle of a trial of labour. This is how, paradoxically, VBAC became more or less associated with home birth assisted by a lay midwife.

It is in such a context that, in 1980, the US National Institute of Health co-sponsored a conference on caesareans.[2] It concluded that VBAC was an appropriate option by which to moderate the climbing rates of caesareans. Widespread interest in trial of labour occurred as a consequence, with a series of studies demonstrating its relative safety.[3,4,5] This is how the rates of successful VBAC in the US increased from 3.4 per cent of women in 1980 to 21.3 per cent in 1991, and to a peak rate of 28.3 per cent of women in 1996.[6] After that the rates started to decline, falling to 16.4 per cent in 2001 and 12.7 per cent in 2002.[7] This decline became more pronounced after the American College of Obstetricians and Gynecologists recommended that a physician be 'immediately available throughout active labor, capable of monitoring labor and performing an emergency cesarean delivery when women undergo a trial of labor after a previous C-section'.[8] The same tendencies and the same fluctuations in the rates of VBAC are currently observed almost everywhere in the world.

A FREQUENTLY ASKED QUESTION

When a woman wants to try to give birth by the vaginal route after a previous caesarean, she first wonders, *what are her chances of having a successful trial of labour*? I have often been surprised by how easy a delivery can be after a previous caesarean for failure to progress or for foetal distress during labour. One of the most typical and exemplary hospital VBAC anecdotes I can mention is about a woman who came to our hospital in the 1970s to give birth to her first baby at the age of 43. After several hours of ineffective contractions, everybody agreed that it was wiser to do a C-section. Two years later, she came back while in hard labour and gave birth quite easily to her second baby by the vaginal route. The second baby was 200 g heavier than the first one. My first out-of-hospital VBAC was the case of a young mother who had expressed her desire to give birth at home to her first baby. However, she finally listened to all the 'wise people' who unanimously commented on the dangers of a home birth for a first baby. After a long labour and failure to progress she needed a caesarean. When her second baby was ready to be born, she decided to trust herself rather than her advisers. She called me one night around 10:00 p.m. while she was not yet in hard labour. I decided to sleep at her home, in a spare bedroom, rather than come and go in the middle of the night. Soon after I arrived, I suddenly woke up when hearing the typical sound of a foetus ejection reflex. One of the plausible interpretations of such easy births is that when a woman has a trial of labour after a previous in-labour caesarean, this implies that she has already had an opportunity to develop her uterine receptors to oxytocin. In other words, the second time her uterus is more sensitive to the effects of the hormone that makes contractions effective.

At the age of evidence-based medicine, we have at our disposal precise data to answer this simple and preliminary question. According to the most authoritative studies, a trial of labour is successful among approximately 70–80 per cent of women.[9,10] Several studies have established predictive scores for the success of such trials, so that women may be given an individualized answer.[11,12,13] Two of these studies used only factors known in pregnancy. The largest one developed a scoring system using also factors known at the time of hospital admission (state of the cervix). The higher the score, the more probable the success of the trial. Rates of successful VBAC ranged from 49 per cent among women scoring 0–2, to 95 per cent among those scoring 8–10. Being young, having also had a prior vaginal delivery and having had a previous caesarean for failure to progress are factors increasing the score. The number of previous caesareans has no significant effect, according to this study.

For obvious reasons these studies could not take into account the degree of privacy, which might be the most important factor for success. Electronic foetal monitoring probably has a strong negative effect that has not been evaluated in the particular case of a VBAC.

A FREQUENT RESPONSE

I have met several women who were in a panic after telling their doctor that they would prefer to try a vaginal delivery in spite of a previous caesarean. The reaction of the doctor was to focus on *the risk of uterine rupture*. After this, some of these women could not get rid of vague and terrifying bloody mental pictures.

Today clinicians are in a position to provide a reassuring and individualized risk assessment. Thanks to a series of recent authoritative studies,[14,15] it is easy to explain that the risk of uterine rupture during a VBAC is in the region of *1 per 200 trials, if the labour has not been induced*. The main risk factor for uterine rupture is induction. According to the largest and most recent study *the risk is multiplied by 15.6 after induction with prostaglandins* and by 4.9 after induction without prostaglandins.[16] Women must also be informed that a rupture can be suspected if there is a failure to progress or if the baby's heart rate is not reassuring. During the intervention, a dehiscence (a 'window') may be found more often than a complete rupture. Women should also be told that uterine rupture is found at a rate of about 0.1–0.2 per cent among women with repeated caesarean without labour.[17,18]

Other factors than labour induction can influence the risks. Maternal age is one of them: the results of two studies suggest that the risks might be increased in women older than 35.[19,20] A fever following caesarean might also increase the risks.[21] Several studies revealed that the risks are increased if the interval between the two births is less than 18 months.[22] Single-layer uterine closure became more popular recently after the publication of several series demonstrating better short-term outcomes, shorter operating times and a shorter stay in hospital. However, the issue of subsequent VBAC has not been addressed. The only 'randomized' trial (the valuable method) was too small (145 women) to detect one real uterine rupture. [23] The results of a larger non-randomized study suggest that a single layer might increase the risks. [24] According to a still more recent study, it is only the risk of uterine windows that is increased.[25] My intuition as a surgeon makes me think that we should also compare interrupted with continuous sutures: in general, whatever the nature of the tissue, interrupted single-layer sutures are followed by good-quality scars.

It is noticeable that until now researchers have not tried to find out if the risks of rupture are higher or lower after a non-labour caesarean. That is why, during my visit to the Suleymaniye Maternity Hospital in Istanbul, I was highly interested in the work of Dr Yazilioglu and Dr Sonmez. They use a technique of ultrasound imaging to evaluate the quality of the uterine scar. They found that the quality of the scar is much better if the caesarean had been performed when the cervix had already reached a certain degree of dilation. The differences were so significant that they now dilate the cervix when performing an elective caesarean and they are in the process of evaluating this new approach.

ANOTHER FREQUENTLY ASKED QUESTION

Mothers who have had a previous caesarean also need to evaluate *the risks for their baby*. A Canadian study can provide answers to their questions. The researchers looked at the outcomes of a series of 2,233 trials of labour after caesarean. In this series one newborn baby died and three suffered a degree of brain damage.[26] According to one of the large studies by the Cambridge–Scotland team, the rate of 'delivery-related perinatal death' among 15,515 women who had a trial of labour was 12.9 per 10,000.[27] This is apparently an acceptable risk. However, we must bear in mind that this number was approximately eleven times greater than the risk associated with planned repeated caesarean. We must carefully scrutinize such data and think in terms of ratio of benefits to risks. To discuss the issue of VBAC it is important to keep in mind the statistical data. Many mothers are able to take into account both statistical data and what they can perceive by intuition.

IN PRACTICE

In the age of the low-segmental technique, the safety of a trial of labour after a previous caesarean is usually underestimated. Doctors and women must just keep in mind that labour should not be induced and that, in general, drugs should not be used. In fact the main risk for the baby is not a uterine rupture:

according to another large study by the Cambridge–Scotland team, in the case of a previous caesarean, the risk of unexplained stillbirth from 39 weeks is double the risk of death related to uterine rupture.[28] This data suggests that another benefit of planned repeat caesarean at 39 weeks may be to reduce the risk of unexplained stillbirth. However, if we think in terms of ratio of benefits to risks, this is not a sufficient reason to refuse a trial of labour and to routinely plan a caesarean at 39 weeks.

The strategy I adopted in the past is still valid in the current scientific context. Even if I was pretty sure that a second caesarean was needed (for example, a misshapen pelvis after an accident), I tended to wait for the first signs of labour and to perform an *in-labour non-emergency caesarean*. This was a guarantee that the baby had given a signal and that mother and baby had started releasing a specific cocktail of hormones. In the usual situation when the trial can continue, the strategy may be simple and easy to summarize. The basic needs of the labouring woman must be met (to feel secure without feeling observed): if the progress of labour is straightforward, the vaginal route is deemed possible; if not, another caesarean should be performed. Most women can give birth by themselves after a previous caesarean when the need for privacy is understood.

15 IF A CAESAREAN BECOMES NECESSARY FOR YOU

Every year, a caesarean is considered the best option for millions of women. The curiosity of some of them is understandable – they ask many practical questions in advance and expect many details. Others don't want to hear these details, simply because they have a precise, preconceived script of what the birth will be like and they cannot imagine that their baby and themselves will be better off with a 'birth from above'. Others have listened to a friend or relative who gave an account of her operation. The following notes are for those who are trying to visualize what is supposed to happen just before, during and just after the operation, should a caesarean become necessary.

FROM CONSENT FORM TO ABDOMEN PAINTING

Whatever the hospital, you are always asked to sign a consent form. The procedures that are necessary before a caesarean can be performed are not always carried out in the same order. It varies from hospital to hospital, depending on the type of anaesthesia used and on whether it is a scheduled section, an in-labour non-emergency section, or a race between the medical team and the progress of a foetal distress. Your abdomen and your pubic hair are shaved. An intravenous drip is inserted and a catheter is installed so that the bladder remains constantly empty and therefore small and less vulnerable. The series of routine procedures also includes a blood pressure cuff placed on your arm. It is also routine to take off any jewellery, apart from the wedding ring. Anaesthetists usually prefer non-emergency situations in order to have the time to focus on what might appear to be details. For example, they may remove your make-up or nail varnish so that changes in colour during the operation can be detected; they will check the implantation of your teeth; they will check that your contact lenses have been removed, etc.

If you already have an epidural in place, it will be topped up. Otherwise, you will be asked to lie on your left side and curl up into a ball, or to sit on the side of the table with your feet on a stool and your elbows resting on your knees. A small area of your back will be painted with antiseptic solution before a needle is inserted between two vertebrae, either for an epidural or, more probably, for a spinal anaesthesia. A spinal takes less time to be effective. Gradually you will feel your legs and abdomen go numb and lose sensation. If you are having a general anaesthetic, the drug will be injected into the intravenous drip and within seconds you will be asleep. As soon as you are asleep and your muscles are relaxed, the anaesthetist will pass a tube down your throat into your trachea in order to protect your lungs and to control the breathing movements.

Whatever the choice of anaesthesia, there will be a time when a nurse will paint the skin of your abdomen with an antiseptic solution. Next the skin is covered with drapes and sterile plastic. The drapes will be put over a bar above your chest so that you cannot see the operation itself.

WHEN THE SURGEON APPEARS

The obstetrician is assisted by one or two helpers, while a nurse and often a paediatrician are present to welcome the baby. Today the father, or a friend or relative, or a doula (lay woman) may be introduced into the operating room (wearing surgical gown, mask and boots).

You may feel tugging or pressure as the baby is pulled from your uterus, but you should not feel pain. In the case of a regional anaesthetic, you are usually presented with your baby during the operation. You might even be able to cuddle with the baby against your shoulder with a bit of assistance. After this, at the very time when the uterus is put back into the abdomen, some women have reported a slight pain, if the surgeon has preferred to exteriorize the uterus for the repair.

As during any abdominal operation, the blood may stagnate in the veins of the legs and pelvis. It is routine to try to prevent the formation of a clot (a deep vein thrombosis) because a part of the clot can travel to the vessels of the lungs. Although such a pulmonary complication is extremely rare today after a fast caesarean, it is important not to scorn well-established protocols. As soon as possible after the operation, you'll be encouraged to move your legs and to walk around your bed. I have adopted the practice of bandaging the legs with special elastic material while the mother is still on the operating table. Furthermore, in the case of overweight women with varicose veins, in the early 1970s I adopted the use of the 'Slendertone' during the operation. Thanks to this electric stimulator, the muscles of the legs never stop contracting and therefore pumping the blood back to the heart.

The time you'll spend in the recovery room and the time you'll spend in the ward depend mostly on the politics of the hospital.

After a caesarean, most women do not need painkillers if the surgical team has gently used hand-held retractors only. One of the main preoccupations during the first days should be that the skin-to-skin contact between you and your baby is disturbed as little as possible.

Back home … to a new family unit.

16   WHAT MOTHERS SAY

We could fill libraries with what women have to say about their experiences of giving birth, via one route or the other.

My role is not to report what women feel. Countless mothers have already done that. When Sarah Clement, a caesarean mother, was preparing her book *The Caesarean Experience*, 200 women completed questionnaires and gave written accounts of their experiences and feelings.[1] Michele Moore, a doctor and caesarean mother, and Caroline de Costa, an obstetrician and the mother of seven, also illustrated their book about caesarean section with first-hand accounts.[2] It is easy to find stories of caesarean births on specialized websites. Many of these sites are American (for example, www.birthlove.com) but there are some non-English-language sites (for example, www.elistas.net/lista/apoyocesareas, a Spanish-language site).

LIMITLESS DIVERSITY

I personally heard countless oral comments on caesarean births in a great diversity of historical and cultural contexts. It is difficult to compare the point of view of an Algerian villager whose baby was rescued by emergency caesarean in the 1950s and the point of view of a London career woman who has chosen to schedule an elective caesarean at the dawn of the twenty-first century. It is difficult to compare the point of view of a Moroccan woman with the point of view of a Brazilian woman. The former does not consider herself a 'real woman' as long as she has not given birth 'from below'. The second one belongs to a 'pro-caesarean culture', where giving birth 'from above' may be regarded as a status symbol. The more we listen to what mothers say, the more we are aware of the limitless diversity of the caesarean experience.

Even in the very frequent, almost standardized situation of an emergency caesarean after a long labour and failure to progress, the way mothers feel will vary depending on so many factors that the emotional reactions may be mostly negative, or mostly positive. For example, for some women it is the end of a dream, a disappointment or the sign of a deficiency. On the other hand, a similar scenario may be experienced in a positive way. As reported in Sarah Clement's book, a mother said: 'When someone mentioned a caesarean as a possibility, it was the light at the end of the tunnel – the only way to finish what I was drowning in the middle of.' Obviously, in this case the caesarean was perceived and welcomed as a rescue operation. In similar circumstances I heard women claiming afterwards that they could not get rid of the feeling that having a caesarean is like 'cheating'. These women are among those who will do all they can to give birth vaginally to their next baby. After giving birth vaginally, they become the happiest and the most vocal of all mothers. In *Silent Knife*, the historical book by Nancy Wainer Cohen and Lois Estner,[3] and in the collection of birth stories published by Lynn Baptisti Richards,[4] VBAC mothers describe feeling 'whole', 'normal', 'female once more', 'strengthened' and 'healed'.

SUPERLATIVES

Most books collecting birth stories are more or less specialized, in the sense that all the births have something in common. For example, it is a series of vaginal births after a caesarean section, or it is a series of births that occurred in the same maternity unit.[5] That is why the book by Sylvie Donna is unique. Written by the mother of three children born in three different environments, it is based on stories of births in a great diversity of contexts. It makes comparisons possible and can help to draw general conclusions.[6] It confirms many word-of-mouth stories. In general, only women who gave birth vaginally by themselves need *superlatives* when recalling their experience of childbirth. My mother used to say that the day of my birth was the most joyful day of her life.

These anecdotes do not contradict scientific studies. Researchers from Melbourne interviewed 272 women at the end of their pregnancy who were expecting their first baby.[7] The interviews were associated with tests evaluating self-esteem and mood. They repeated the interviews and tests after birth. Those women who had a spontaneous vaginal delivery were more likely to experience a marked improvement in mood and an elevation of self-esteem across the late pregnancy to the period following birth. Those who had a caesarean, on the other hand, were more likely to experience deterioration in mood and a diminution of self-esteem. A study like this should be repeated in a pro-caesarean cultural milieu such as Shanghai or São Paulo, for example. Measuring self-esteem is measuring love of oneself. Mothers raise questions about the future of love.

17   THE PERINEAL
PREOCCUPATION

The perineal preoccupation is central in the debate about 'à la carte caesarean'.

Among the many female obstetricians who prefer a scheduled caesarean for the birth of their own babies, four out of five indicated the risk of perineal damage as their main preoccupation.[1] In general the fear of vaginal rupture appears to be an important component of the fear of labour.

The medical term 'prophylactic caesarean' often refers to a caesarean in which one of the objectives is to prevent pelvic floor disorders that can lead to urinary and anal incontinence, reduced sexual sensitivity, and organ prolapse.

In the age of caesarean on demand the debate must be put into perspective. The risks of urinary incontinence and faecal incontinence among women who gave birth by the vaginal route are real and well-documented.

PUBLISHED FACTS

According to a Norwegian evaluation based on an inquiry among more than 15,000 women belonging to the same community the risk of stress urinary incontinence is 12.2 per cent among women who gave birth vaginally versus 6.9 per cent among those who had caesareans, and 4.7 per cent among those who never had babies.[2] The protective effect of caesarean delivery has been confirmed in the case of twin births and multiple births in general.[3]

Women rarely talk spontaneously about anal incontinence. However, a survey among 242 women who gave birth vaginally (without an obvious tear of the anal sphincter) revealed that twelve of them developed anal incontinence, including loss of flatus (wind accumulated in the bowels), which lasted longer than twelve months.[4] Similar results were obtained from an inquiry among 1,667 women who had previously given birth in one hospital over a six-month period. Six per cent of them reported faecal incontinence related to the present or a previous childbirth.[5]

From the abundant literature about perineal damages after childbirth, we can conclude that, from that point of view, *the most dangerous scenario is a forceps delivery following a long, arduous labour.* This is the main lesson of a British study about tears involving the anal sphincter. More than 8,000 women who had given birth vaginally were included in the study.[6] It is now well-established that an episiotomy does not prevent this sort of tear and that a ventouse (vacuum) is not as dangerous for the perineum as forceps. This is also the main lesson of an Australian study that investigated the effect of childbirth on pelvic organ mobility thanks to an ultrasound technique (translabial ultrasound).[7] They measured in particular the bladder neck descent when the woman is asked to forcibly breathe out while keeping the mouth and nose closed. The mean bladder neck descent is spectacular after a forceps delivery (14.5 mm), compared with vacuum (9 mm), normal vaginal delivery (7.2 mm), caesarean during the second stage (4 mm) and caesarean during the first stage (2.6 mm).

Anal incontinence after childbirth is now being studied from several new perspectives. Nerve injuries are being evaluated via electromyographic studies that can demonstrate processes of denervation and renervation of the sphincter.[8] An ultrasound technique (anal endosonography) revealed that, after the birth of a first baby, 35 per cent of mothers have detectable sphincter defects.[9]

INTERPRETATIONS

These hard data need to be tempered. First, according to the Norwegian evaluation, the protective effect of caesarean on urinary incontinence dissipates by age 50, so that older women have the same rate of urinary incontinence regardless of the way they gave birth. Furthermore, in terms of perineal damage and anal physiology, the protective effect of caesarean delivery is pronounced only if the operation is performed before a dilatation of 8 cm.[10]

More importantly, all these studies have been performed in large conventional hospitals. In such environments the basic needs of labouring women are usually ignored and the physiological processes are highly disturbed.

THE FOETUS EJECTION REFLEX

The more I try to combine what I have learnt from my experience of hospital births and home births, the more I am convinced that the best way to protect the perineum and to avoid a serious tear is to deviate as little as possible from the physiological model. In other words, to create the conditions for an authentic foetus ejection reflex.[11,12]

I am often asked to clarify the difference between the foetus ejection reflex and the reflex induced by the pressure of the baby's head (or buttocks) on the perineal muscles.[13] A real foetus ejection reflex can occur long before the descent of the presenting part, or long after. It can start before complete dilation or after complete dilation. Usually it does not occur at all because the prerequisite is complete privacy. I am familiar with this 'reflex', in the context of home birth, when I follow the progress of labour from another room through the sound the woman is making, while her husband/partner goes shopping, and when there is nobody else around other than an experienced, motherly, *silent* and low-profile doula. I cannot remember many cases of authentic 'reflex' in the presence of the baby's father. During the 'reflex' there is a short series of irresistible, uncontrollable contractions, with no room for voluntary movements; the labouring woman can be in the most unexpected postures (often asymmetrical, bending forward).

I have interpreted this reflex as the effect of a sudden spectacular reduction in the activity of the neocortex (the thinking brain), making possible the release of a complex hormonal cocktail. The release of high levels of hormones of the adrenaline family is suggested by the sudden expression of fear (often a very short episode of fear of death)[14] that precedes the irresistible contractions, and by a sudden tendency to grasp something and to be upright. The most helpful thing to do in terms of facilitating the foetus ejection reflex is just to interpret this sudden expression of fear ('Kill me ... Let me die', etc.) without interfering: reassuring rational words – a stimulation of the neocortex – would inhibit the reflex. The release of a high peak of oxytocin is of course suggested by the sudden power and efficiency of the uterine contractions.

We must keep in mind that the term 'foetus ejection reflex' was originally used by Niles Newton when she was studying the factors influencing the birth of mice,[15] that is, mammals who do not have a neocortex as powerful as ours. The 'reflex' can occur among humans on condition that the activity of the neocortex is dramatically reduced, so that the human handicap is overcome. Another opportunity to refer to the 'animal power of birth'.

I learnt from a powerful foetus ejection reflex induced by a cup of champagne. This was around 1980 in the Pithiviers hospital. A woman in not-yet-hard labour was in a double bedroom. Her roommate, who was already celebrating the birth of her baby, gave her a cup of champagne. The unexpected effect was a sudden series of so powerful contractions that the second mother's baby was born on the way to the birthing room. My interpretation was that the bubbles speeded up the absorption of alcohol, so that there was an immediate effect on brain activity that other sorts of wine cannot have. Anyway, the capacity champagne has to release inhibitions has been widely tested, whenever the goal is to create an erotic or not-too-formal atmosphere. Recently I met Dominique Marquette, a home birth midwife and a native of Epernay, the famous wine centre in the area of Champagne. When preparing for a home birth, she always suggests that the family keeps a bottle of champagne in the fridge, officially to celebrate the birth afterwards. In fact, now and then, in precise circumstances, she offers a glass of champagne to the woman in labour in order to release inhibitions. I mention these anecdotes in order to interpret and illustrate the nature of this reflex. The conclusion is not that labouring women should be routinely offered a glass of champagne!

I have never had to repair the perineum after a real undisturbed foetus ejection reflex. One of the many reasons probably is that in such a context the mother is more often than not bending forward, for example, on hands and knees. In such postures, the mechanism of vulva opening is different from that of other postures. First the anterior part of the vulva opens more quickly; then the deflexion of the head tends to be delayed and, when the face is coming out, the chin is more lateral. I use this opportunity to mention that, if by chance there is a benign tear (usually because there has been no authentic foetus ejection reflex) I do not stitch it. If the mother does not spread her legs at all during the first two weeks (avoiding looking at the perineum, avoiding the lotus posture, etc.) the cicatrization will be perfect.

One of the advantages of the term foetus ejection reflex incidentally is to underline the similarities between the different episodes in our sexual life. As Niles Newton pointed out,[16] in the milk ejection reflex, the sperm ejection reflex and the foetus ejection reflex there is always a sudden explosive release of oxytocin. This release of oxytocin is always highly dependent upon environmental factors.

Today, if we focus on the perineal preoccupation, a policy of scheduled caesarean at term may be considered well-founded only as long as the conditions for a foetus ejection reflex are not understood, and as long as only twentieth-century criteria are taken into account. It is quite another matter if we introduce twenty-first-century criteria, particularly if we accept that the scientification of love[17] is one of the most vital aspects of the current scientific revolution.

18   EITHER ... OR ...

FUTURISTIC STRATEGIES

For those who have learnt the preliminary lessons about the scientification of love, and for those who have acquired the capacity to think in terms of civilization, the basis of the future strategies are obvious. *The aim should be that as many women as possible give birth vaginally thanks to an undisturbed flow of love hormones.*

However, the primary objective should not be to reduce the rates of caesareans: it would be dangerous, if not preceded by a first step. This first step should be an attempt to promote a better understanding of birth physiology and particularly a better understanding of the basic needs of women in labour. In hospitals where the watchword is to reduce the rates of caesareans, the first effect is usually an increased number of difficult births by the vaginal route and of dangerous last-minute emergency caesareans. This is exactly what we should avoid in the age of the safe caesarean. I have had many recent reports of deliveries during which the obstetrical team tried 'everything' in order to avoid a caesarean: drip of synthetic oxytocin, epidural anaesthesia and, finally, either a forceps delivery with episiotomy or even a caesarean after trying the use of forceps. Forceps have their place in museums. The last time I used forceps was in February 1965.

We previously mentioned the many reasons why elective caesareans should also be avoided as far as possible. When a non-labour caesarean has been scheduled there is no guarantee that the baby – particularly its lungs – are perfectly mature. Maternal and foetal hormones associated with the progress of labour contribute to achieve the maturation of the lungs. The increased risks of respiratory problems are well documented. In general a non-labour caesarean implies that the foetus has not participated in the initiation of labour. It also implies that the foetus has not been given the opportunity to put into action its system of stress hormones. Breastfeeding difficulties are more probable than after an in-labour caesarean. Furthermore the chances for a successful vaginal birth after caesarean seem to be better in the case of an in-labour caesarean.

Finally we must start to prepare for a binary strategy, with *two basic scenarios. Either* the birth process is straightforward by the vaginal route. In spite of several generations of medicalized birth, this will become more common on the day when the importance of privacy and the reason for authentic midwifery are rediscovered. *Or* the birth process does not appear as straightforward. This should lead to an in-labour non-emergency caesarean. The point is to decide early enough during the first stage of labour when a caesarean is indicated. We need new tests adapted to twenty-first-century strategies. Scores associating a great number of criteria have recently been designed in order to try to detect early on in the birth process those women who are destined to have a caesarean.[1]

THE BIRTHING POOL TEST

The birthing pool test is the typical example of a tool adapted to futuristic strategies. It is based on a simple fact. When a woman in hard labour enters the birthing pool and is immersed in water at body temperature, a spectacular progress in the dilation is supposed to occur within an hour of two. If the already well-advanced dilation remains stable in spite of water immersion, privacy (no camera!) and dim light, one can conclude that there is a major obstacle. There is no reason for procrastination. It is wiser to perform an *in-labour non-emergency caesarean* immediately.

Up to the mid-1970s I had used what I called lumbar reflexotherapy, in precise circumstances, as a test in order to try to decide as early as possible if a caesarean is necessary. The technique is simple. One or two intracutaneous injections of sterile water are made in the back, on each side of the spine, at the level of the muscular depression that is just below the last rib. The point is to create tiny pimples, like those produced by the sting of a nettle.[2] This reflexotherapy is efficient when the dilation has reached 5 cm and only when the contractions are felt as lumbar pains. When the lumbar pains have gone, only a discomfort above the pubic bone continues while cervical dilation is progressing. When the dilation does not progress, it means that there is probably a major mechanical obstacle.

After we had introduced a birthing pool in our maternity unit in the late 1970s I tended to forget the use of lumbar reflexotherapy.

In the early 1980s, I had already mentioned in a mainstream medical journal[3] the reason why we originally introduced the concept of birthing pools in the Pithiviers hospital. I had also described the most typical scenario:

> We tend to reserve the pool for women who are experiencing especially painful contractions (lumbar pain, in particular), and where the dilatation of the cervix is not progressing beyond about 5 cm. In these circumstances, there is commonly a strong demand for drugs. In *most cases*, the cervix becomes fully dilated within 1 or 2 hours of immersion ...'

At that time I could only refer to *most cases*. Afterwards, I analysed the outcomes in the rare cases when the dilation had not progressed after an hour or two in the bath. I realized that finally a caesarean had always been necessary, more often than not after long and difficult first and second stages. This is how I started tacitly to take into account what I had not yet called the birthing pool test.

More recently it happened that I mentioned the birthing pool test during information sessions for doulas. This is how I learnt from a series of reports about births in London hospitals. It is obvious that many long and difficult labours, with the usual range of drugs preceding an emergency caesarean, would be avoided if the birthing pool test had been interpreted. One of these anecdotes is particularly significant. A woman in hard labour arrived in a maternity unit with her doula while the dilation of the cervix was already well advanced. Soon after, she entered the birthing pool. More than an hour later the dilation had not progressed. The doula – who was aware of the birthing pool test – was adamant that this woman could not safely give birth by the vaginal route. A senior doctor was eventually called and diagnosed a brow presentation. A brow presentation is difficult to diagnose in early labour and is incompatible with the vaginal route. In this case the doula knew that a caesarean would be necessary, although she could not explain why.

The birthing pool test implies that an internal exam has been performed just before immersion so that, if necessary, a comparison will become possible after an hour or two. This is an important practical detail, because midwives who are familiar with undisturbed and unguided births in silence, semi-darkness and privacy can usually follow the progress of labour with criteria other than a repeated evaluation of the dilation of the cervix.

INTERPRETATIONS

Today we can offer a physiological scenario explaining why immersion in water at body temperature makes the *contractions more effective during a limited period of time*. When a woman enters the pool in hard labour there is immediate pain relief and therefore an immediate reduction in the levels of stress hormones. Since stress hormones and oxytocin are antagonistic, the main *short-term response* is usually a peak of oxytocin and therefore a spectacular progress in the dilation.

After that there is a long-term complex response, which is a redistribution of blood volume. This is the standard response to any sort of water immersion. There is more blood in the chest.[4] When the chest blood volume is increased, certain specialized cells in the atria release a sort of hormone commonly called ANP (Atrial Natriuretic Peptide) that interferes with the activity of the posterior pituitary gland.[5] We can all observe the effects of reduced activity of our posterior pituitary gland after being in a bath for a while: we pass more urine. This means that the release of vasopressin – the water retention hormone – is reduced. In fact the chain of events is not yet completely clarified in the current scientific context.[6] We have recently learnt that oxytocin – *the love hormone – has receptors in the heart(!)* and that it is a regulator of ANP.[7]

In practice, we just need to remember that the immediate peak of oxytocin following immersion in warm water will induce a feedback mechanism and eventually the uterine contractions will become less effective after an hour or two.

SIMPLE RECOMMENDATIONS

In general, all the recommendations that should be widely divulged regarding the use of the birthing pool are based on this double response to water immersion.

The first practical recommendation is to give a great importance to the time when the labouring woman enters the pool. Experienced midwives have many tricks at their disposal to help women to be patient enough so that they can ideally wait until 5 cm dilation. A shower, that more often than not implies complete privacy, is an example of what the midwife can suggest while waiting. A survey published in the *British Medical Journal* clearly indicated that many women stay too long in the bath. One reason is that many of them enter the bath long before they are dilated 5cm.[8]

The second recommendation is to avoid planning a birth under water. When a woman has planned a birth under water she may be the prisoner of her project; she is tempted to stay in the bath while the contractions are getting weaker, with the risk of long second and third stages. There are no such risks when a birth under water follows a short series of irresistible contractions. In general women should avoid a precise, preconceived script of what the birth of their baby will be like.

Let us add a simple *recommendation regarding the temperature*. It is easy to check that the water temperature is never above 37°C (the temperature of the maternal body). Two cases of neonatal deaths have been reported after immersion during labour in prolonged hot baths (39.7°C in one case).[9] The proposed interpretation was that the foetuses had reached high temperatures (the temperature of a foetus is 1°C higher than the maternal temperature) and could not meet their increased needs in oxygen. The foetus has a problem with heat elimination.

At the dawn of a new phase in the history of childbirth one can anticipate that, if a small number of simple recommendations are taken into account, the use of water immersion – in the case of difficult labour – can seriously compete with the use of drugs, particularly epidural anesthesia and synthetic oxytocin. Then helping certain women to be patient enough and enter the pool at the right time will appear as a new aspect of the art of midwifery, and as *an attempt to increase the number of women who release a flow of love hormones while giving birth.*

PAM ENGLAND

Pam England is the author of the influential book *Birth from Within*. About a week after giving birth to her son Luc at home, in New Mexico, Pam felt the need to express the animal power of birth. This is how she painted *The Lion Roars in Labor*. Her first child had been born by caesarean. In 1984, after her caesarean delivery, she came to France and visited me in Pithiviers. She recently commented on our conversation and on the birth of her children:

> The few hours we spent together in Pithiviers, October of 1984 changed my life forever, and years later, the simple advice you gave me while I was carrying the 'cub' in the painting was perfect. After telling you my cesarean story with my first labor, I asked you for advice on bringing about a normal birth the second time. You thought for a moment and said, 'Lock yourself in the bathroom and don't let anyone in, not even the midwife. You will be alright.' That is all you said. At the time I remember thinking, 'That's it! That's your advice? I just told you my traumatic birth story and am freaked out and that is all you have to say?'

I trusted you. I followed your advice (just short of locking myself in the bathroom), I cocooned myself in the Dark Feminine (which is represented by the dark colors in the lower half of the painting). The midwife did exactly what I asked her to do: Nothing. In the absence of any interference at all, I felt-my-way instead of thought my way through the process; it was like being blindfolded in a labyrinth where one can't get lost and must 'feel' one's way, and be determined to get to the center.

Like so many women, I was over-educated yet unprepared for labor the first time. Still, having a cesarean birth was a great Teacher for me; but I knew I did not complete the 'lesson'. The second time I became pregnant, I took seriously what you teach women to do: I forgot everything I knew about labor and birth. I entered my Lucy-brain, I entered the Divine Feminine and abandoned all hope and all control (in the painting, the primal life force surging through me is represented by the white zig zag line). When I was pushing Luc out I arched my back and 'roared'; I felt then I embodied the ferocity of a roaring lion. Luc was born minutes later. Birthing normally at home was the completion of the 'lesson of birth' I took birth for; and I have never been the same.

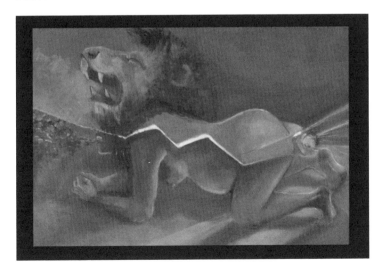

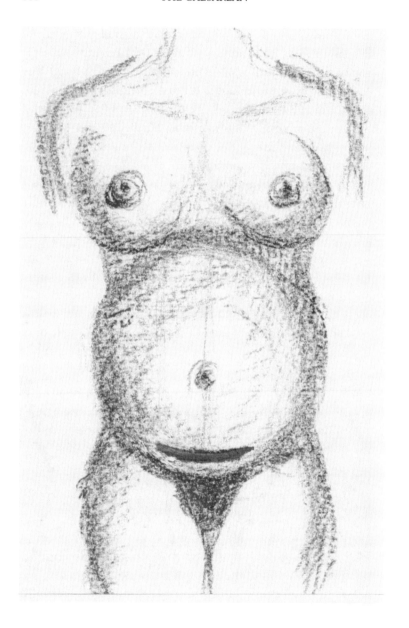

Or ... from above.

19   ANTENATAL SCARE

Let us imagine that one of the main public health preoccupations is to make sure that as many women as possible can give birth vaginally thanks to an undisturbed flow of love hormones. Let us imagine that there is also an agreement on the futuristic 'either–or' strategy, based on a better understanding of birth physiology.

We must first think short-term and wonder what changes might be introduced immediately.

It is well understood that the prerequisite for labour to establish itself properly is a low level of anxiety. In other words, the more a pregnant woman is subjected to anxiety-provoking stimuli, the more difficult the birth process will be. A low level of anxiety is also the prerequisite for optimal growth and development of the baby in the womb. The preliminary practical questions must therefore focus on what can influence the emotional state of pregnant women. Everybody has heard of women who were unsettled and apprehensive after an antenatal visit. It is obvious that the dominant style of antenatal care – constantly focusing on potential problems – has an inherent 'nocebo effect'. The nocebo effect is a negative effect on the emotional state of pregnant women and indirectly of their families. It occurs whenever a health professional does more harm than good by interfering with the imagination, the fantasy life or the beliefs of a patient or a pregnant woman.[1,2,3]

IN AN IDEAL WORLD

In an ideal world, the main *preoccupation of doctors* and other health professionals involved in prenatal care should be *to protect the emotional state of pregnant women*.

It should not take so long for an adaptable health professional to shift towards a positive attitude and to overcome any current habits. Modern pregnant women cannot be blissfully happy. All of them have at least one reason to be worried: 'Your blood pressure is too high or too low', 'Your weight is increasing too quickly or too slowly', 'You are anaemic', 'You might haemorrhage because your platelet count is low', 'You have gestational diabetes', 'Your baby is too small or too big', 'There is too much liquid around the baby', 'There is a lack of liquid', 'The placenta is low', 'You are 18 and teenage pregnancy is associated with specific risks', 'You are 39 and older-age pregnancy is associated with specific risks', 'Your baby has not yet turned head first', 'The baby's back is on the right side, which makes the birth difficult', 'According to the blood sample you are at risk of having a Down's syndrome baby', 'You did not take folic acid at the right time and we must consider the risk of spina bifida', 'You are not immunized against rubella', 'You are Rh negative', 'If you have not given birth on Wednesday, we must consider an induction', etc. Is it still possible to be a 'normal' woman?

In the same ideal world, the expectant mother should be *guided by a primary practical question: 'What can the doctor do for me and my baby?'* If we consider the usual case of a woman who knows that she is pregnant and who knows roughly when her baby was conceived, *the humble response should be: 'Not a lot, apart from detecting a gross abnormality and offering an abortion'.*

TOWARDS THE END OF *ROUTINE* MEDICALIZED PRENATAL CARE?

In many countries about ten prenatal visits is routine. In other words, most women have ten opportunities to hear about potential problems. At each visit a battery of tests is offered. These traditional patterns of medical care are based on the belief that more antenatal visits mean better outcomes. They are not based on scientific data. That is why the very concept of routine medicalized care and the number of visits must be re-examined.

British studies failed to find any association between beginning prenatal care late and adverse outcomes for the mother or the baby[4] or between the number of visits and the onset of the disease eclampsia.[5] This casts doubts on the efficacy of such protocols. Within the British National Health Service, the number of visits is not as strongly associated with socio-economic status as it is in the US. This makes the results of the British studies comparatively easier to interpret than those of the American studies.[6,7]

However, it is worth analysing a 2002 report by the Centers for Disease Control and Prevention in the US. It appears that women who were born outside the US are more likely than their racial and ethnic counterparts born in the US to begin prenatal care late or to have no prenatal care at all. 'In spite of this' (or perhaps 'because of this'?) American-born women are more likely than their counterparts born outside the US to give birth preterm or to give birth to a low-weight baby. It is also fruitful to analyse trials comparing different schedules of antenatal visits. One was conducted in California, in the Kaiser Permanente Medical Center.[8] A second trial, in southeast London, involved 2,794 women.[9] A third one, by the World Health Organization, involved 53 centres in Thailand, Cuba, Saudi Arabia and Argentina.[10] None of these trials demonstrated any benefits of conventional schedules compared with reduced visit schedules.

One may also wonder if women who have a great number of antenatal visits give birth more easily than those with none. A study on the effect of cocaine use on the progress of labour unexpectedly suggested the opposite.[11] The researchers took into account that one-third of cocaine users had no prenatal care. It was therefore essential to determine the average dilation at admission among non-users of cocaine who had no prenatal care. It appeared that the mean dilation at admission in this group was more than 5 cm.

THE CONTENT OF ANTENATAL VISITS RECONSIDERED

Not long ago the main reason for the first antenatal visit was *to establish the diagnosis of pregnancy* and to determine the due date. Since reliable pregnancy tests can now be bought over-the-counter, most women have their pregnancy confirmed before visiting a health professional and have a reliable date of conception. Knowing that a pregnancy lasts about nine months, most women can calculate the most probable time for the birth of their baby. One can therefore claim that the primary reason for an early antenatal visit has disappeared.

Routine ultrasound scanning in pregnancy became the symbol of modern prenatal care. It is also its most expensive component. A series of studies compared the effects on birth outcomes of routine ultrasound screening versus the selective use of the scans. An American trial involved more than 15,000 pregnant women.[12] The last sentence of the article is unequivocal: 'The findings of this study clearly indicate that ultrasound screening does not improve perinatal outcome in current US practice.' Around the same time, an article in the *British Medical Journal* [13] assembled data from four other comparable trials. The authors concluded:

> Routine ultrasound scanning does not improve the outcome of pregnancy in terms of an increased number of live births or of reduced perinatal morbidity. Routine ultrasound scanning may be effective and useful as a screening for malformation. Its use for this purpose, however, should be made explicit and take into account the risk of false positive diagnosis in addition to ethical issues.

It is possible that, in the future, a new generation of studies (in the framework of Primal Health Research) will cast doubts on the absolute safety of repeated exposure to ultrasound during foetal life. One of the effects of selective use is to reduce dramatically the number of scans, particularly in the vulnerable phase of early pregnancy.

Even in a high-risk population of pregnant women, ultrasound scans are not as useful as commonly believed. Evidence from several trials suggests that sonographic identification of foetal growth retardation does not improve outcome despite increased medical surveillance.[14,15] In diabetic pregnancies it has been demonstrated that ultrasound measurements are not more accurate than clinical examination in identifying high-birth-weight babies.[16] This led to the memorable title of an editorial of the *British Journal of Obstetrics and Gynaecology*: 'Guess the weight of the baby'.

In many countries, the amount of red blood cells pigment (*haemoglobin concentration*) is routinely measured in pregnancy. There is a widespread belief that this test can effectively detect anaemia and iron deficiency. In fact, this test cannot diagnose iron deficiency because the blood volume of pregnant women is supposed to increase dramatically, so the haemoglobin concentration indicates first the degree of blood dilution, an effect of placental activity. A large British study, involving more than 150,000 pregnancies,[17] found that the highest average birth weight was in the group of women who had a haemoglobin concentration between 8.5 and 9.5.

Furthermore, when the haemoglobin concentration fails to fall below 10.5 there is an increased risk of low birth weight, preterm birth and pre-eclampsia. The regrettable consequence of routine evaluation of haemoglobin concentration is that, all over the world, millions of pregnant women are wrongly told that they are anaemic and are given iron supplements. There is a tendency both to overlook the side effects of iron (constipation, diarrhoea, heartburn, etc.) and to forget that iron inhibits the absorption of such an important growth factor as zinc.[18] Furthermore, iron is an oxidative substance that can exacerbate the production of free radicals and might even increase the risk of pre-eclampsia.[19]

Another routine screening practised in certain countries is for so-called gestational diabetes. This is the reason for using the *glucose tolerance test*. If the glycaemia (amount of glucose in the blood) is considered too high after absorption of sugar, the test is positive. This diagnosis is useless because it merely leads to simple recommendations that should be given to all pregnant women, such as: avoid simple sugars (including soft drinks, sodas, etc.), choose complex carbohydrates (pasta, bread, rice, etc.), and take a sufficient amount of physical exercise. A huge Canadian study demonstrated that the only effect of routine glucose tolerance screening was to inform about 3 per cent of pregnant women that they had gestational diabetes.[20] The diagnosis did not change the birth outcomes.

Even the routine *measurement of blood pressure* in pregnancy may be reconsidered. Its original purpose was to detect the preliminary signs of pre-eclampsia, particularly at the end of a first pregnancy. But increased blood pressure, without any protein in the urine, is associated with good birth outcomes.[21, 22,23,24] The prerequisite for the diagnosis of pre-eclampsia is the presence of more than 300 mg of protein in the urine per 24 hours. Finally, it is more useful to rely on the repeated use of the special strips for urinalysis one can buy in any pharmacy. Measuring the blood pressure is thus not essential.

After challenging the very principle of routine medicalized care in pregnancy and after evaluating the content of antenatal visits, we can explore the issue from a third perspective. We can wonder *what the doctor can do* after the conception of a baby in order to influence outcomes. Since prematurity is a major preoccupation, let us focus on what medical care can offer in order to reduce the incidence of preterm births. Recently, considerable research focused on the potential for antibiotic prophylaxis. A large trial involving more than 6,000 women did not support the use of antibiotics.[25] Furthermore, the treatment of vaginal infection in early pregnancy does not decrease the incidence of preterm delivery.[26] Surgical closure of the cervix (cerclage) has been widely used in order to reduce the risk of premature birth especially in cases of a short and 'incompetent' cervix. In fact, the data conflict about the value of this technique which reportedly doubles the risk of fever after the birth of the baby.[27] Medical interventions also do not reduce the risk of having a small-for-date baby. Even bed-rest restrictions have been shown to be useless and even harmful.

THE FUTURE

At the same time, when we have the data exposing routine medicalized prenatal care as a huge waste of time and money, we are constantly pressured *to focus on what can be done before conception.* Today it is beyond doubt that prevention of abnormalities such as spina bifida is effective before conception; almost everybody has heard about folic acid. In terms of nutrition we emphasized the facts revealed by comparing the Danish study and our own studies of fish consumption. An important Danish study found that the risk of having a premature or a low-birth-weight baby was much higher among women who never eat fish, compared to those who eat fish regularly, at least once a week.[28] There is an apparent contradiction between the Danish results and the results of our own studies. After encouraging a series of pregnant women to eat sea fish, we could not detect any significant effect of our dietary recommendations in the perinatal period in terms of birth weight and duration of pregnancy (apart from an increased head circumference).[29] The point is that the Danish researchers assessed dietary habits that preceded to a great extent the beginning of pregnancy. It is probable that dietary recommendations in antenatal clinics occur too late to have detectable effects in the perinatal period.[30,31]

An accumulation of data provided by a great variety of medical disciplines indicates what should be considered the main threat for the health of the unconceived generations: the intrauterine pollution by synthetic fat soluble chemicals that accumulate over the years in human adipose tissues. The foundation of any preconceptional programme such as our 'accordion method' must be to reduce the body burden of synthetic pollutants before conceiving a baby.[32] The same issue concerns the father-to-be since the development of the concept of male-mediated developmental toxicity: it appears today that certain diseases or developmental disorders occur more frequently when the man has been exposed to certain pollutants.

We should not conclude that there is no need at all for

medical visits in pregnancy: it is almost impossible to make a comprehensive list of all the reasons why women might need the advice or the help of a qualified health professional before giving birth. It is the word 'routine' that should be discarded. It is easy to explain why the current habits are a waste of time and money; it is also easy to explain why they are potentially dangerous. It is dangerous to misinterpret the results of a routine test and to tell a healthy pregnant woman that she is anaemic and that she needs iron supplements. It is dangerous to present an isolated increased blood pressure measurement as bad news. It is dangerous to tell a pregnant woman that she has 'gestational diabetes'.

The fall of routine medicalized antenatal care should go hand-in-hand with a rediscovery of the basic needs of pregnant women. We cannot dissociate the physiological changes in pregnancy and birth physiology. It is as if the birth process was physiologically prepared long in advance. We must pay attention to a study demonstrating that, during pregnancy, there is a significant reduction of the blood flow in the large arteries going to the brain.[33] Is the pregnant woman preparing herself to reduce the activity of her neocortex in order to make the birth possible?

One of the needs of pregnant women is to socialize and share their experiences. It is easy to create occasions for that: swimming, yoga, prenatal exercise sessions … I well remember the atmosphere of happiness that accumulated during singing encounters in the maternity unit at the Pithiviers Hospital in France. These singing sessions probably had more positive effects on the development of babies in the womb and also on the birth process than a series of ultrasound scans.[34]

20   RECEIVED IDEAS

It is easy and there is an urgent need to challenge many received ideas that translate and transmit a deep-rooted lack of understanding of the basic needs of women in labour. Some of them originated in natural childbirth circles. Others originated in medical circles. All of them contribute to reducing the number of women who can give birth while releasing a flow of love hormones.

YOU NEED ENERGY!

It is commonplace to compare labouring women with athletes who are advised to consume large amount of carbohydrates, protein and fluids before starting extreme physical exertion.[1] Authors of articles about nutrition during labour have suggested that we should learn from sports medicine.[2] Many birth attendants are influenced by these comparisons and encourage women to eat food such as pasta at the onset of labour, and drink something sweet when labour is established: 'You need energy!'

These ideas about nutrition are in contradiction with our current understanding of the physiology of labour. When the first stage is progressing, it is a sign that low levels of the hormones of the adrenaline family are kicking in. A low level of adrenaline and good progress in the first stage imply that the *skeletal (voluntary) muscles are at rest*. Relaxation and low levels of adrenaline are almost synonymous. When a birth is as physiological as possible, the labouring woman has a tendency to be immobile during the first stage. When all the skeletal muscles are at rest, such as when the mother is lying on her side or is on all fours, the energy expended is slight and the need for carbohydrates is minimal, insofar as glucose is the favourite fuel of skeletal muscles.

When labour is progressing easily, it is also a sign that *the neocortex* – the part of the brain so highly developed among humans – *is at rest*. The neocortex is the other organ of the human body whose primary fuel is glucose. Finally, while the skeletal muscles and the neocortex tend to reduce their activity, there are only two parts of the body which are really active: the uterine muscle, and the primitive part of the brain, that is to say the old small structures shared with all the other mammals (hypothalamus, pituitary gland), whose role is to release the hormones involved in the birth process.

The energy expenditure of the primitive part of the brain is insignificant. As for the uterine muscle, it is a smooth (involuntary) muscle. Smooth muscles are between 20 and 400 times more energy-efficient than skeletal muscles. Furthermore, they can easily use fatty acids (rather than glucose) as a fuel. Because the body stores large amounts of fat, in practice there is no risk of fuel shortage for the smooth muscles. It is essential to understand that smooth muscles, and occasionally skeletal muscles, use fatty acids as a fuel. The observations by Paterson and colleagues are highly significant.[3] In order to explain their importance, we must recall that when there are ketone bodies in the urine, it simply means that fatty acids have been used as a fuel. They found that ketone levels were higher in women who had been starved for twelve hours before an elective caesarean under general anaesthesia than they were for women who had been in labour. This confirms that *labouring women spend less energy than those who are only waiting for an operation without being in labour.*

Comparing labouring women to marathon runners is misleading and potentially dangerous. The side effects of sugar during labour are well-documented.[4] Birth attendants should know that pure sugars tend to lower the pain threshold.[5] Moreover, there is evidence that when the mother has been given an infusion containing glucose, the intensity of jaundice in the newborn baby is greater.[6] Physiologists can explain why.

Comparing a labouring woman with a marathon runner can lead to other mistakes, such as overestimating the need for water. It has been written that the considerable amount of water lost during labour needs to be replenished in order to prevent dehydration and its consequences. In fact, labouring women don't lose a great amount of water because their level of pituitary water-retention hormone (vasopressin) is high and because their skeletal muscles are not active. When labour starts, the body is 'waterlogged' and the real risks are those of water intoxication and low levels of sodium in the blood.[7,8] A full bladder is another price to pay for the marathon analogy.

These theoretical considerations need to be confronted with what we can learn by interpreting the behaviour of labouring women. For several decades, either in a hospital or at home, I have learned from thousands of women who were neither encouraged nor discouraged to eat and drink in labour. Although there are always exceptions, it is possible to summarize several simple rules. The *first point* is that labour rarely starts when a pregnant woman is hungry. This makes sense since hunger tends to increase the level of hormones of the adrenaline family. *Second*, when labour is really well-established women do not eat, so that I have serious doubts that a woman is actually in labour if she is eating. Labour is a difficult diagnosis. When a woman has contractions every five minutes and is told that her cervix is 1 or 2 cm dilated, she understands that undoubtedly she is in labour. But this diagnosis is the cause of many so-called long labours, with the accompanying increased risk of intervention that is preceded by the use of drugs. When a woman actually needs to eat, it means that she needs some food for active labour to establish itself. In fact, many women go to the hospital in prelabour, but labour cannot establish itself as long as the level of adrenaline has not been lowered, thanks to an ingestion of food. *The third thing* that I have learned is that women who feel really free and have not been told that they need 'energy' usually drink water rather than sweet fluids. They often have an urgent need to sip water just before the last irresistible contractions of the foetus ejection reflex (a sign of a sudden release of adrenaline).

We must recall that eating and drinking have been prohibited in many hospitals for many years in order to prevent potentially fatal complications of general anaesthesia when the stomach if full (solid regurgitations can obstruct the airway and acid regurgitations and aspiration can lead to serious pneumonitis). Today, at a time when most caesareans are performed under spinal or epidural anaesthesia, we are in a position to under-stand that, when there are no restrictions, the balance of benefits to risks is positive and the rate of intervention is reduced. It is significant that the only case of aspiration at the North Central Bronx Hospital (New York) for ten years hap-pened during the six months when restrictions on eating and drinking were imposed.[9] It is also significant that in the Netherlands, where 30 per cent of the births occur at home (women having free and constant access to the refrigerator), the maternal mortality rate is less than 10 per 100,000, and the rate of caesarean around 10 per cent.

Even if there is a renewed interest for birth physiology in the near future, we will still have to accept that a woman's *nutritional needs during labour are too complex to be managed* by a birth attendant. Generally speaking, labour cannot be managed. Women must rely on what they feel, rather than on what they read or what they were told. To encourage a woman to eat noodles or to add honey to her tea is not more appropriate than it is to impose restrictions. The only recommendation we can make is to avoid making recommendations.

YOU MUST WALK!

Once I was in the house of a woman in prelabour. Her husband and I were sharing a meal in the kitchen. Suddenly the mother-to-be appeared. She told me, as if imploring a favour: 'I am tired.' I just said: 'If you are tired, go to bed and lie down.' She was surprised by such a simple suggestion. As many other women, she had been told or she had read that walking and using the force of gravity would make the labour easier. This simplistic vision is not new. As early as 1833, William DeWees wrote that 'the preposterous custom of obliging her [the labouring woman] to walk the floor with a view to increase the pains when tardy should be peremptorily forbidden'.[10]

Once more the widespread tendency to 'manage' labour is based on a lack of understanding of birth physiology and of the basic needs of women in labour. When a labouring woman does not feel the need to stand up and to walk, it is a good sign. It means that her level of adrenaline is probably low. This is the prerequisite for an easy labour. During the first stage of an easy and fast birth, women are often passive; for example, on all fours or lying down. To suggest any sort of muscular activity at that phase can be counter-productive, even cruel. It is true that in physiological conditions, when the woman does not feel observed or guided, she often has a sudden tendency to be more vertical during the irresistible last contractions of the foetus ejection reflex.[11]

Some women want to hang from something or somebody. Others suddenly stand up, often leaning forwards against a piece of furniture. Others, who are kneeling, have a sudden tendency to lift their body. This is related to a sudden and transitory rush of adrenaline.[12]

This belief that a woman in labour should walk is widespread in the natural childbirth movement and in medical circles as well. This is how we can explain the popularity of the term 'walking epidural' and also the publication in the most prestigious medical journals of studies trying to evaluate the effect of walking on labour and delivery. Of course, none of the studies conducted with a reliable method (randomized trials with a large enough numbers of participants) could demonstrate any effect.[13,14,15] It is significant that, in the most authoritative of these studies, 22 per cent of the women who were assigned to walking stayed in bed.[16] It is the hormonal balance that is important. In the case of an unmanaged birth, the position of the mother is a consequence of the hormonal balance.

YOU NEED SUPPORT!

The terms 'support', 'emotional support' and 'supportive companion' are ubiquitous. They proliferate in books about 'natural childbirth'. They proliferate in the titles of articles published in the mainstream medical literature.[17,18,19,20,21,22,23,24,25] The word 'support' suggests that a woman cannot give birth by herself: she needs some energy brought by another person. This word suggests an active role for the birth attendant. It belongs to the depowering vocabulary commonly used in the field of childbirth.

In order to realize how misleading and therefore noxious is the fashionable vocabulary, we must once more refer to the basic needs of labouring women. A woman in labour needs to feel secure without feeling observed or judged. This is the prerequisite for a reduction of the activity of her neocortex, the thinking brain. An analogy between falling asleep and 'falling in labour' may be useful.[26] In both cases the neocortex must be at rest and the basic needs are the same. Let us think of a little girl who needs to feel the presence of her mummy at bedtime. She needs to feel secure without feeling observed or judged. A mother would never say 'My young daughter needs a support person to fall asleep.' Another opportunity to recall that an authentic midwife is first and foremost a mother-figure.

Not only is the term 'support' misleading, furthermore it is harmful. It has overshadowed the basic mammalian need for privacy. An anecdote may be useful to make clear why it can be dangerous. A home-birth midwife was telling her colleagues about a birth that had been unexpectedly long and difficult. She could not understand why, because this woman had 'a lot of support': 'She had a very supportive husband; her old friend Jenny was very supportive as well; so was her doula' ... I guess this woman would have given birth easily if there had been no one in the house except an experienced and silent midwife.

The term 'support' became overused after the publication by the team of John Kennell and Marshall Klaus of an important study conducted in the 1970s in Guatemala. In two busy hospitals where 50–60 babies are born every day and where doctors and nurses trained the American way had established the routines, they evaluated the effects on statistics of the presence of a lay woman (a 'doula') belonging to the community. They found that the presence of a doula reduces dramatically the incidence of all sorts of intervention and the use of drugs, and tends to improve the outcome. The term 'supportive companion' was introduced in the title of the report.[27] The researchers reproduced their study in Houston, Texas, in a neighbourhood where the population is predominantly Hispanic and incomes are low. The birthing caregivers there were directed by English-speaking residents in a twelve-bed ward. The doulas were mothers who could speak Spanish. As in Guatemala, the presence of a doula had obvious positive effects.[28] The authors once more used the word 'support' in order to interpret the results. My own interpretation is that, in such an unfamiliar and strange environment, the *doula* is felt to be a protector. She is as protective as a mother would be. She is a *screen* between the labouring women and the white-coat staff.

Interestingly, these results were not confirmed by studies conducted in middle-class American populations. We must underline that in such a different context the participation of the baby's father is considered normal.[29] There has even been an (expensive!) study involving nearly 70,000 women and their babies in 13 US and Canadian hospitals.[30] The objective was to evaluate the 'effectiveness of nurses as providers of birth labor support'. Specialized nurses had received 'formal training in labor support techniques'. The conclusions were that continuous labour support 'does not affect the likelihood of cesarean delivery or other medical or psychosocial outcomes of labor and birth'. This study confirms that 'labouring women don't need support'.[31] They need to feel secure without feeling observed.

It is urgent to reconsider a vocabulary that translates and dangerously transmits the current deep-rooted lack of understanding of birth physiology.

THE FRUITS ON THE TREE

According to the traditional wisdom in rural Western Europe, a baby in the womb should be compared to a fruit on a tree. All the fruits on the same tree are not ripe at the same time. A fruit that has been caught before being ripe will never be very fit to eat and will quickly go bad. It is the same with a baby.[32,33] In other words it is well-accepted that some babies need a much longer time than others before they are ready to be born.

Modern pregnant women, on the other hand, are given a very precise due date. The pregnancy is punctuated by routine medical visits according to an established programme. At the age of medicalized prenatal care, the duration of pregnancy is more precisely calculated in weeks rather than in months. Long in advance, women are warned that if the baby is not born at a certain date, the labour will be induced. The first effect of such attitudes is that in many hospitals more than a quarter of the births are artificially induced. The other effect is that more and more women doubt that they are able to make the labour start without the help of doctors.

An induced labour is more difficult than a labour that started spontaneously. It usually leads to the need for epidural anaes-thesia and drip of oxytocin, more often than not preceding a cascade of intervention, such as ventouse (vacuum), forceps or emergency caesarean. The labour induction epidemic contrib-utes to explaining the rising rates of caesareans all over the world.

At the root of this epidemic are statistics. When looking at very large numbers of births, it is clear that the outcomes are optimal when the baby is born between 38 and 40 weeks. The statistics are not as good when focusing on babies born at 41 weeks or after. Such data lead to simplistic conclusions: 'If we routinely induce the labour whenever the pregnancy lasted more than a certain number of weeks (41 in many hospitals), we'll eliminate the risks of foetal distress and even deaths related to post-maturity.' The risk of death related to post-maturity is not a legend, but it is usually overestimated. It should be balanced with all the risks associated with induction. Is it wise to induce a quarter of labours, in order to save one baby out of thousands? Are more selective strategies possible? The answer is yes.

In order to gradually replace the dominant strategies, the analogy of the fruits on a tree is perfectly relevant. All the fruits are not mature on the same day. It is the same with babies. We should favour an *individualized and selective approach*. I know from personal experience that such an approach is realistic. The principle is simple. After a certain date (for example 41 weeks) the condition of the baby is assessed *on a day-to-day basis*. As long as the baby is in good shape, it is possible to wait. From the time when the daily assessments have started, only the wellbeing of the baby is taken into consideration, whatever the duration of pregnancy. The most common scenario by far is that one day the labour starts spontaneously and a healthy baby is born. When the newborn baby is pealing, it means that it was already post-mature.

Several methods can be combined in order to check that the foetus is not in danger. For a pregnant woman it is easy to evaluate on a day-to-day basis the frequency of the movements of the baby in the womb. When there is a dramatic change overnight, this should be considered a warning. For the medical staff, on the other hand, it is easy to repeat clinical exams and ultrasound scans. As long as there is a sufficient amount of liquid in the uterus, it is almost a guarantee that the baby is not in danger. We are at a time when most women are offered a great number of useless ultrasound scans all along their pregnancy: these scans are useless compared with what an experienced practitioner can expect from a clinical exam after listening to the mother-to-be. It seems, on the other hand, that many doctors are paradoxically reluctant to repeat scans in the period surrounding birth and even when the baby might be overdue. This is precisely the time when scans provide precious data that have huge practical implications. An individualized strategy might also lead to the more frequent use of hormonal assessments after the so-called due date.

And what if, suddenly, the baby seems to be in danger before the labour starts? From my point of view, in this case, it is wiser to perform a caesarean right away. The priority is to avoid a risky last-minute emergency intervention. With such a strategy, labour induction will finally be exceptionally rare and the number of caesareans related to post-maturity will be much lower than if all labours were induced at 41 weeks.

One of the drawbacks of the current dominant strategies is that many women don't spend the last days of their pregnancy in peace. They are obsessed by the date they were given for induction, if the labour has not started spontaneously. They are in an emotional state that probably tends to delay the onset of labour. Some of them try to use non-medical methods of induction. They don't always realize that any effective method (from acupuncture to sexual intercourse) implies that the labour starts before the baby has given a signal of its maturity. Some methods are undoubtedly unpleasant and even dangerous. This is the case with the use of castor oil.

Eliminating the received ideas that are at the root of such practices would be the first step towards an increased number of births involving a cocktail of love hormones.

21 THE FUTURE OF THE MIDWIFERY–OBSTETRICS RELATIONSHIP

Humanity has to face an unexpected challenge. At the beginning of the twenty-first century a great proportion of the world population does not use the vaginal route to be born. The time has come to try to anticipate the probably enormous effects on the characteristics of our civilizations of such a sudden turning point in the history of childbirth.

Meanwhile, we must aim at starting to increase the proportion of women who give birth to their baby and its placenta, compared with those who are delivered by the medical institution. In the framework of short-term objectives, we have already considered the reasons to help pregnant women to live in peace, by reducing the degree of antenatal scare induced by the nocebo effect of a certain style of medical visits. We have also considered the need to eliminate widespread received ideas.

AN INEVITABLE LONG-TERM OBJECTIVE

The difficult and inevitable long-term objective is to reconsider the midwifery–obstetrics relationship. The key is to understand the reason for midwifery and to rediscover authentic midwifery. With the perspective and the language of physiologists we can easily explain that a labouring woman needs to feel secure without feeling observed or judged. This leads us to understand the midwife as a mother-figure and as a substitute for the mother: in an ideal world, our mother is the prototype of the person with whom one feels secure without feeling observed or judged. This also leads us to understand the limits of the role of the medical institution. In general, the role of doctors is not to be directly involved in physiological processes. Their role is to be the expert in unusual and pathological situations.

International comparisons support the lessons provided by the physiological perspective. Countries with skyrocketing rates of caesareans are those where the obstetricians outnumber the midwives to such a degree that they play the role of the primary caregivers. These countries include in particular Brazil and most Latin American countries, China, Taiwan, South-Korea, India, Turkey, Greece and Italy … On the other hand, countries with good statistics including moderate rates of caesareans are those where the midwives outnumber the obstetricians and remain the primary caregivers. In that group we can include Holland, Sweden and Norway. Countries such as the US, the UK, France, Germany, Japan, Australia and New Zealand are in an intermediate situation.

SMASHING POLITICAL CORRECTNESS

Timorous reforms cannot lead to the reintroduction of a great number of authentic midwives. Radical changes overthrowing the current systems are needed.

The first important issue is *the number of midwives compared with the number of obstetricians* in a given population. The prerequisite for the rediscovery of authentic midwifery is a dramatic reduction in the number of obstetricians. Authentic obstetricians should not have the time to control every birth.

They should appear on demand. Today most obstetricians have a dangerous lack of experience. In the US, for example, the number of obstetricians is in the region of 40,000; for the number of births a year that is in the region of 4,000,000. This implies that a typical obstetrician is in charge of about 100 births a year. The typical American obstetrician has the experience of about one or two twin births a year. They need years of practice to see one real placenta praevia (the baby cannot get out because the placenta is on the way) and a whole career to see one real eclampsia. On the day when they have to do a caesarean for a transverse presentation, they must adapt their technique after referring to textbooks, because it is a rare situation they have probably never met. During the many years when I was in charge of about 1,000 births a year, I had the feeling that it was the right number to maintain sufficient experience. A dramatic reduction in the number of obstetricians must undoubtedly be balanced by an appropriate increase in the number of midwives.

The shift towards authentic midwifery is more than a matter of numbers. *The central and inescapable question should be: 'How do we select women who will become midwives?'* In other words, those who are in charge of midwifery schools should base their criteria on a straightforward question: 'How can we offer the *guarantee* that this particular candidate will be perceived as a mother-figure and that her presence will not disturb labouring women?' Common sense and clinical observation provide a simple answer: the prerequisite for entering a midwifery school should be to be a mother with a personal experience of undisturbed birth with no medication. Let us recall that in most traditional societies a midwife was a mother or a grandmother who had many children. Women who had many children were usually those who had easy births. Such a programme, easy to summarize in one sentence, is bound to face many difficulties and will have to overcome predictable obstacles.

The first major obstacle will be the usual reaction to the idea that an authentic midwife should have a personal experience of giving birth. People live in the present and usually react by claiming that they know wonderful midwives who are not mothers. We all know such midwives. The point is that, in order to prepare for the future, we must learn to think long-term and to think in terms of civilization. It is difficult to understand the need to offer a *guarantee* that cannot be provided by any other mode of selection. I personally dare to guarantee that on the day when all midwives will be mothers having the experience of giving birth without intervention or medication, the current rates of caesareans will be consigned to history.

After decades of industrialized childbirth, there will be another obstacle to adopting these radically new criteria of selection. We must realize that in many countries the number of women with experience of undisturbed vaginal birth is already insignificant. These are precisely the countries where there is an urgent need to develop many midwifery schools and to detect many potentially authentic midwives. In order to break the vicious circle, a policy will be needed that will insistently encourage the rare women who gave birth by themselves to become midwives, at least during a certain phase of their life.

During an inevitable *period of transition*, we must understand the importance of the *doula phenomenon*. Its development, even in countries where there are many conventionally selected and trained midwives, must attract our attention and needs to be interpreted. If the doula is the mother-figure a young woman can rely on during the whole period surrounding birth, the doula phenomenon will become an effective way to hasten the rediscovery of authentic midwifery. If the doula is just another person introduced in the birthing place in addition to the midwife, the doctor and the father, her presence will be counter-productive. If the focus is on the training of the doula rather than on her way of being and her personality, the doula phenomenon will be a missed opportunity.

Since the project of rediscovering authentic midwifery is incompatible with political correctness, I dare to go a step further and raise a complementary question: 'What if the prerequisite for a doctor to become specialized in obstetrics was to be a mother with personal experience of undisturbed vaginal birth?' Good statistics associated with caesarean rates below 10 per cent are not utopian *if* we are lucid enough to smash political correctness.

These considerations about the future of the midwifery–obstetrics relationship may lead to overturning the order of the main preoccupations humanity has to face. Rediscovering authentic midwifery is not yet on the agenda of all those who want to create a positive future.

There are reasons for optimism. A breakthrough scenario is imaginable ... *if* the vital urgency of changing childbirth is recognized outside specialized circles. *If* not ... a breakdown scenario is also imaginable.

22   TOO RATIONAL TO SURVIVE?

The will to survive and the struggle for life are not rational. The desire for descendants and the need to take care of them are not rational. The many facets of love are outside the field of rationality. We survive as individuals, as groups or as a species because we are not purely rational beings.

Rationality is related to the activity of the part of the brain – the new brain or neocortex – that is gigantically developed only among humans. The neocortex appeared originally as a tool at the service of the instincts that are indispensable for the survival of the species. *Homo sapiens* is the only mammal whose neocortex is strong enough to exceed its role as a tool, and often seems to be interfering in activities that are much too complex for its abilities and negligent of its original assignment.

Cultural milieux have always rationalized the different episodes of sexual life. They have channelled and organized sexual attraction and mating through rituals and institutionalized marriage. They always had a tendency to socialize and to ritualize childbirth and the initiation of lactation. However, this aspect of the domination of nature, which has been the basis of our civilizations for many millennia, has suddenly reached another order of magnitude. We are crossing a threshold.

IS HUMANITY THREATENED BY AN EXCESS
OF RATIONALITY?

Today the conception of a baby appears more than ever as a
rational decision. This has been confirmed by countless sur-
veys, such as the one by Flexecutive, a British recruitment
consultancy, or by the (British) Institute of Public Policy
Research, which commissioned the Lever Fabergi Family Report
2003. Today a woman decides whether or not to have a baby, 'in
the same logical way that she decides whether or not she will
take out a joint mortgage'. Arguments for motherhood are
divided into 'pros' and 'cons'. The pro arguments are easily
pooh-poohed and classified as either indoctrinated thinking ('I
will not be a complete woman until I am a mother') or teenager
logic ('If I love my baby, it will love me', or 'I will have a real live
doll').

   This shift towards a human being more dominated by
rationality occurs at the very time when the development of
electronics and computer technology offers powerful tools that
prolong and reinforce the activity of the neocortex. Today we
may utilize artificial intelligence. Until now the reason for most
tools had been to potentiate or to replace the functions of the
limbs. We invented all sorts of vehicles for what was originally
the function of our legs. Levers and cranes are powerful
substitutes for our arms.

   Furthermore, this shift occurs at the very time when the
widespread use of the safe caesarean can smash the previous
limits to brain evolution, by making easier the transmission to
future generations of the tendency for larger brain size.

   *A high degree of rationality would not be threatening if it
were balanced by an enhanced development of the capacity to
love* and of the will to live. But it is a tendency towards a

weakened and impaired capacity to love that we are now expecting … *if* the breakdown scenario prevails.

We must attach real importance to data supporting De Catanzaro's evolutionary theory of human suicide,[1] according to which a threshold intelligence is necessary for self-damaging behaviour (an expression of an impaired capacity to love oneself). According to an ecological study comparing 85 countries, the suicide rates are related to the average intellectual development.[2] Furthermore, excess suicide prevalence has been observed in the highly gifted.

Today we must confront the implications of an easy, safe and well-accepted caesarean with the lessons provided by the 'scientification of love'.[3]

We must urgently ask the unaskable:

How does the capacity to love develop?

Can a super-brainy *Homo sapiens* survive without love?

Can humanity survive the safe caesarean?

NOTES AND REFERENCES

CHAPTER 2
ONE ROUTE OR THE OTHER

1 Behague DP, Victoria CG, Barros FC. Consumer demand for caesarean sections in Brazil. *BMJ* 2002; 324: 942–5.
2 Tranquilli AL, Garzetti GG. A new ethical and clinical dilemma in obstetric practice: caesarean section on 'maternal request'. *Am J Obstet Gynecol* 1997; 177: 245–6.
3 Harer W. Patient choice cesarean. *Am Coll Obstet Gynecol Clin Review* 2000; 5: 2.
4 Controversies: should doctors perform an elective caesarean section on request? *BMJ* 1998; 317: 463.
5 Wagner M. Choosing caesarean section. *Lancet* 2000; 356: 1677–80.
6 Nygaard I, Cruikshank DP. Should all women be offered elective cesarean delivery? *Obstet Gynecol* 2003; 102(2): 217–19.
7 Al-Mufti R, McCarthy A, Fisk NM. Survey of obstetricians' personal preference and discretionary practice. *Eur J Obstet Gynecol Reprod Biol* 1997; 73: 1–4.
8 Gabbe SG, Holzman GB. Obstetricians' choice of delivery. *Lancet* 2001; 357: 722.
9 Steer P. Caesarean section: an evolving procedure? *Brit J Obstet Gynecol* 1998;105: 1052–5.
10 Stein R. Elective caesareans judged ethical. *Washington Post*, 31 October 2003: A32.

CHAPTER 3
SAFER AND SAFER

1 Kerr JMM. The technique of cesarean section, with special reference to the lower uterine segment incision. *Am J Obstet Gynecol* 1926; 12: 729–34.

2 Pfannenstiel JH. Uber die Vorteile des suprasymphysaren fascien-querschnitts fur die gynakologische koliotomien zugleich ein bei-trag zu der indikationsstellung der operationswege. *Samml Klin Vortr Gynakolog* (Leipzig) 1900; 97: 1735–56.

3 Joel-Cohen S. *Abdominal and Vaginal Hysterectomy: New Techniques Based on Time and Motion Studies.* William Heinemann Medical Books, London 1972.

4 Stark M, Finkel AR. Comparison between the Joel-Cohen and Pfannenstiel incisions in cesarean section. *Eur J Obstet Gynecol Reprod Biol* 1994; 53(2): 121–2

5 Tulandi T, Al-Jaroudi D. Non closure of peritoneum: a reappraisal. *Am J Obstet Gynecol* 2003; 189(2): 609–12.

6 Wallin G, Fall O. Modified Joel-Cohen technique for caesarean delivery. *Brit J Obstet Gynaecol* 1999; 106: 221–6.

7 Hannah ME, Hannah WJ, Hewson SA, et al. Planned caesarean section versus planned vaginal birth for breech presentation at term: a randomised multicentre trial. *Lancet* 2000; 256: 1375–83.

8 The European mode of delivery collaboration. Elective caesarean-section versus vaginal delivery in prevention of vertical HIV-1 transmission: a randomized clinical trial. *Lancet* 1999; 353: 1035–9.

9 Krebs L, Langhoff-Roos J. Elective cesarean delivery for term breech. *Obstet Gynecol* 2003; 101(4): 690–6.

10 Harper MA, Byington RP, Espeland MA, et al. Pregnancy-related death and health care services. *Obstet & Gynecol* 2003; 102(2): 273–8.

11 Fenton PM, Whitty CJM, Reynolds F. Caesarean section in Malawi: prospective study of early maternal and perinatal mortality. *BMJ* 2003; 327: 587–90.

12 Pereira C, Bugalho A, et al. A comparative study of caesarean deliveries by assistant medical officers and obstetricians in Mozambique. *Brit J Obstet Gynaecol* 1996; 103: 508–12.

CHAPTER 4
BREAKING A VICIOUS CIRCLE

1. Varner MW, Fraser AM, et al. The intergenerational predisposition to operative delivery. *Obstet Gynecol* 1996; 87(6): 905–11.

CHAPTER 5
WHEN OUR DREAMS COME TRUE
Further reading

This B. *La requête des enfants a naître*. Le Seuil, Paris 1982.

Young J. *Caesarean Section: The History and the development of the operation from earliest times*. HK Lewis, London 1944.

Pundel J. *Histoire de l'opération césarienne. Etude historique de la césarienne dans la médecine, l'art et la littérature, la religion et la législation*. Presses Académiques Européennes, Bruxelles 1969.

Sue P. Essais historiques, littéraires et critiques sur l'art des accouchements. *Fac Med* Paris No. 34678, 1779.

Wyman A L. The female practitioner of surgery. *Medical history* 1984; 28: 22–41.

CHAPTER 6
TOWARDS A SUPER-BRAINY HOME SAPIENS?

1 Odent M. *Primal Health*. First edition, Century-Hutchinson, London 1986. Second edition, Clairview, Forest Row, West Sussex 2002.

2 Odent M. Prématurité et créativité, in *Les cahiers du nouveau-né no. 6. Un enfant, prématurément*. Le Vaguerese ed. Stock, Paris 1983.

3 English J. *Different Doorway: adventures of a cesarean born*. Earth Heart, Point Reyes Station, CA 1985.

CHAPTER 7
TWENTY-FIRST-CENTURY CRITERIA

1 Odent M. *The Scientification of Love*. Free Association Books, London 1999. Revised edition 2001.

2 Pedersen CA, Prange JR. Induction of maternal behavior in virgin rats after intracerebroventricular administration of oxytocin. *Pro Natl Acad Sci* USA 1979; 76: 6661–5.

3 Russell JA, Douglas AJ, Ingram CD. Brain preparations for maternity: adaptive changes in behavioral and neuroendocrine systems

during pregnancy and lactation. *Progress in Brain Research* 2001;
133: 1–38.

4   Odent M. The early expression of the rooting reflex. *Proceedings of
the 5th International Congress of Psychosomatic Obstetrics and
Gynaecology, Rome 1977*. Academic Press, London 1977: 1117–19.

5   Odent M. 'Colostrum and civilization' in *The Nature of Birth and
Breastfeeding*. First edition, Bergin and Garvey, Westport, CT
1992. Second edition, (*Birth and Breastfeeding*) Clairview, Forest
Row, West Sussex 2003.

6   Odent M. The early expression of the rooting reflex. *Proceedings of
the 5th International Congress of Psychosomatic Obstetrics and
Gynaecology, Rome 1977*. Academic Press, London 1977: 1117–19.

CHAPTER 8
LONG-TERM THINKING

1   Odent M. *Primal Health*. First edition, Century-Hutchinson, London 1986. Second edition, Clairview, Forest Row, West Sussex
2002.

2   Xu B, Pekkanen J, Hartikainen AL, Jarvelin MR. Caesarean section
and risk of asthma and allergy in adulthood. *J Allergy Clin Immunol*
2001; 107(4): 732–3.

3   Xu B, Pekkanen J, Jarvelin MR. Obstetric complications and
asthma in childhood. *J Asthma* 2000; 37(7): 589–94.

4   Kero J, Gissler M, Gronlund MM, Kero P, Koskinen P, Hemminki
E, Isolauri E. Mode of delivery and asthma – is there a connection?
Pediatr Res. 2002 July; 52(1): 6–11.

5   Bager P, Melbye M, Rostgaard K, Stabell Benn C, Westergaard T.
Mode of delivery and risk of allergic rhinitis and asthma. *J Allergy
Clin Immunol* 2003 Jan; 111(1): 51–6.

6   McKeever TM, Lewis SA, Smith C, Hubbard R. Mode of delivery
and risk of developing allergic disease. *J Allergy Clin Immunol* 2002
May; 109(5): 800–2.

7   Faxelius G, Hagnevik K, Lagercrantz H, Lundell B, Irestedt I.
Catecholamine surge and lung function after delivery. *Arch Dis
Child* 1983: 58(4): 262–6.

8   Hook B, Kiwi R, Amini SB, Fanoroff A, Hack M. Neonatal
morbidity after elective repeat cesarean section and trial of labour.
Pediatrics 1997; 100: 348–53.

9 Eggesbo M, Botten G, Stigum H, et al. Is delivery by cesarean section a risk factor for food allergy? *J Allergy Clin Immunol* 2003; 112(2): 420–6.

10 Hay D, Pawlby S, Angold A, et al. Pathways to violence in the children of mothers who were depressed postpartum. *Dev Psychol* 2003; 39: 1083–94.

11 Tinbergen N, Tinbergen A. *Autistic children*. Allen and Unwin, London 1983.

12 Hattori R, et al. Autistic and developmental disorders after general anaesthetic delivery. *Lancet* 1991; 337: 1357–8.

13 Hultman C, Sparen P, Cnattingius S. Perinatal risk factors for infantile autism. *Epidemiology* 2002; 13: 417–23.

14 Zwaigenbaum L, Szatmari P, et al. Pregnancy and birth complications in autism and liability to broader autism phenotype. *J Am Acad Child Adolesc Psychiatry* 2002; 41: 572–79.

15 Lord C, Mulloy C, et al. Pre- and perinatal factors in high-functioning females and males with autism. *J Autism Dev Disord* 1991; 21(2): 197–209.

16 Wilkerson DS, Volpe AG, et al. Perinatal complications as predictors of infant autism. *Int J Neurosci* 2002; 112(9): 1085–98.

17 Iuul-Dam N, Townsend J, Courchesne E. Prenatal, perinatal and neonatal factors in autism, pervasive developmental disorders, and the general population. *Pediatrics* 2001; 107(4): E63.

18 Courchesne E, Carper R, Akshoomoff N. Evidence of brain overgrowth in the first year of life in autism. *JAMA* 2003; 290: 337–44.

19 Green L, Fein D, et al. Oxytocin and autistic disorder: alterations in peptides forms. *Biol Psychiatry* 2001; 50(8): 609–13.

20 Odent M. Between circular and cul-de-sac epidemiology. *Lancet* 2000; 355: 1371.

CHAPTER 9
TOWARDS AN UNPRECEDENTED CULTURAL DIVERSITY?

1 Marais EN. *The Soul of the White Ant*. Methuen, London 1937.

2 Krehbiel D, Poindron P. Peridural anaesthesia disturbs maternal behaviour in primiparous and multiparous parturient ewes. *Physiol Behav* 1987; 40: 463–72.

3 Lundbland EG, Hodgen GD. Induction of maternal-infant bonding

in rhesus and cynomolgus monkeys after caesarian delivery. *Lab Anim Sci* 1980; 30: 913.

4   English J. *Fingers Pointing to the Moon*. Earth Heart, Point Reyes Station, CA 1999.

5   Finger C. Brazilian beauty. *Lancet* 2003; 362: 1560.

CHAPTER 10
ENTERING THE WORLD OF MICROBES

1   Cederqvist LL, Ewool LC, Litwin SD. The effect of foetal age, birth weight, and sex on cord blood immunoglobulin values. *Am J Obstet Gynecol* 1978 Jul 1; 131(5): 520–5.

2   Coe C, Levine S, Rosenberg LT. Effects of age, sex and psychological disturbance on immunoglobin levels in squirrel monkey. *Developmental Psychobiology* 1988; 21(2): 161–75.

3   Dubos R. Staphylococci and infection immunity. *Am J Dis Child* 1966; 105: 643–45.

4   Eggesbo M, Botten G, Stigum H, et al. Is delivery by cesaren section a risk factor for food allergy? *J Allergy Clin Immunol* 2003; 112(2): 420–6.

5   Odent M. Future of BCG. *Lancet* 1999; 354: 2170.

6   Feinmann J. A culture of hype? *The Times* 26 Nov 2003, T2, 8.

CHAPTER 11
ENTERING THE WORLD OF ODOURS

1   Odent M. The early expression of the rooting reflex. *Proceedings of the 5th International Congress of Psychosomatic Obstetrics and Gynaecology, Rome 1977*. Academic Press, London 1977: 1117–19.

2   Sarnat HB. Olfactory reflexes in the newborn infant. *J Pediatr* 1978; 92: 624–6.

3   Axel R. The molecular logic of smell. *Sci Am* Oct 1995: 130–7.

4   Marchini G, Lagercrantz H, Winberg J, Uvnas-Moberg K. Foetal and maternal plasma levels of gastrin, somatostatin and oxytocin after vaginal delivery and elective cesarean section. *Early Human Development* 1988; 18(1): 73–9.

5 Brennan P, Kaba H, Keverne EB. Olfactory recognition: a simple memory system. *Science* 1990; 250: 1223–6.

6 Sullivan RM, Zyzak DR, Skierkowski P, Wilson DA. The role of olfactory bulb norepinephrine in early olfactory learning. *Develop Brain Research* 1992; 70: 279–82.

7 Varendi H, Christensson K, Porter RH, Winberg J. Soothing effect of amniotic fluid smell in newborn infants. *Early Hum Dev* 1998 Apr 17; 51(1): 47–55.

8 Varendi H, Porter RH, Winberg J. Attractiveness of amniotic fluid odor: evidence of prenatal olfactory learning? *Acta Paed* 1996 Oct; 85(10): 1223–7.

9 Schaal B, Marlier L, Soussignan R. Olfactory function in the human foetus: evidence from selective neonatal responsiveness to the odor of amniotic fluid. *Behav Neurosci.* 1998 Dec; 112(6): 1438–49.

10 Marlier L, Schaal B, Soussignan R. Neonatal responsiveness to the odor of amniotic and lacteal fluids: a test of perinatal chemosensory continuity. *Child Dev* 1998 Jun; 69(3): 611–23.

11 Sullivan RM, Toubas P. Clinical usefulness of maternal odor in newborns: soothing and feeding preparatory responses. *Biol Neonate* 1998 Dec; 74(6): 402–8.

12 Cernoch JM, Porter RH. Recognition of maternal axillary odors by infants. *Child Dev* 1985 Dec; 56(6): 1593–8.

CHAPTER 12
NURSING THE CAESAREAN BORN

1 Csontos K, Rust M, Hollt V, et al. Elevated plasma beta-endorphin levels in pregnant women and their neonates. *Life Sci* 1979; 25: 835–44.

2 Akil H, Watson SJ, Barchas JD, Li CH. Beta-endorphin immunoreactivity in rat and human blood: Radioimmunoassay, comparative levels and physiological alterations. *Life Sci* 1979; 24: 1659–66.

3 Rivier C, Vale W, Ling N, Brown M, Guillemin R. Stimulation in vivo of the secretion of prolactin and growth hormone by beta-endorphin. *Endocrinology* 1977; 100: 238–41.

4 Nissen E, Uvnas-Moberg K, Svensson K, Stock S, Widstrom AM, Winberg J. Different patterns of oxytocin, prolactin but not cortisol

release during breastfeeding in women delivered by caesarean section or by the vaginal route. *Early Human Development* 1996; 45: 103–18.

5 Zanardo V, Nicolussi S, Giacomin C, Faggian D, Favaro F, Plebani M. Labor pain effects on colostral milk beta endorphin concentrations of lactating mothers. *Biology of the Neonate* 2001; 79(2): 79–86.

6 Odent M. The early expression of the rooting reflex. *Proceedings of the 5th International Congress of Psychosomatic Obstetrics and Gynaecology, Rome 1977*. Academic Press, London 1977: 1117–19.

7 Odent M. *Birth and Breastfeeding*. Clairview, Forest Row, West Sussex 2003 (British edition of *The Nature of Birth and Breastfeeding*. Bergin and Garvey, USA 1992).

8 Lundell BP, Hagnevik K, Faxelius G, Irestedt L, Lagercrantz K. Neonatal left ventricular performance after vaginal delivery and cesarean section under general or epidural anesthesia. *Am J Perinat* 1984; 1(2): 152–7.

9 Hagnevik K, Faxelius G, Irestedt L, Lagercrantz K, Lundell BP, Persson B. Catecholamine surge and metabolic adaptation in the newborn after vaginal delivery. *Acta Paediatr Scand* 1984; 73(5): 602–9.

10 Christensson K, Siles C, et al. Lower body temperatures in infants delivered by caesarean section than in vaginally delivered infants. *Acta Paediatr* 1993; 82(2): 128–31.

11 Lie B, Juul J. Effect of epidural vs. general anesthesia on breastfeeding. *Acta Obstet Gynecol Scand* 1988; 67: 207–9.

12 Almeida JAG. *Breastfeeding: A Nature–Culture Hybrid*. Editora Fiocruz, Rio De Janeiro 2001.

13 Brasil/MS, 2000. *Prevalencia do Aleitamento Materno nas Capitals Brasileiras e no Distrito Federal*. Relatorio Preliminar, Versao 3, Brasilia, Ministerio da Saude.

14 Marques NM, Lira PI, da Silva NL, et al. Breastfeeding and early weaning practices in northeast Brazil: longitudinal study. *Pediatrics* 2001; 108(4): E66.

15 Shawky S, Abalkhail BA. Maternal factors associated with the duration of breastfeeding in Jeddah, Saudi Arabia. *Paediatr Perinat Epidemiol* 2003; 17(1): 91–6.

16 Martin J. *Infant Feeding 1975: attitudes and practice in England and Wales*. OCPS Social Survey Division, HMSO, London 1978.

17 Doganay M, Avsar F. Effects of labor time on secretion time and quantity of breastmilk. *Int J Gynaecol Obstet* 2002; 76(2): 207–11.

CHAPTER 13
A THOUSAND AND ONE REASONS TO BE OFFERED
A CAESAREAN

1 Morris S, Stacey M. Resuscitation in pregnancy. *BMJ* 2003; 327 1277–9.
2 Smith GCS, Pell JP, Dobbie R. Caesarean section and risk of unexplained stillbirth in subsequent pregnancy. *Lancet* 2003; 362: 1779–84.
3 McKenna DS, Ester JB, Fischer JR. Elective cesarean delivery for women with a previous sphincter rupture. *Am J Obstet Gynecol* 2003; 189(5): 1251–6.
4 Hannah ME, Hannah WJ, et al. Planned caesarean section versus planned vaginal birth for breech presentation at term: a randomised multicentre trial. *Lancet* 2000; 356: 1375–83.
5 Odent M. Home breech birth. *The Practising Midwife* 2003; 6(1): 11.
6 Odent M. The foetus ejection reflex. *Birth* 1987; 14: 104–5.
7 Noble E. *Having Twins – and More*. Third edition. Houghton Mifflin, Boston 2003.
8 Ibid.
9 Dominguez K, Lindegren ML, L'Almada PJ, et al. Increasing trend of cesarean deliveries in HIV-infected women in the United States from 1994 to 2000. *J Acquir Immune Defic Syndr* 2003; 33(2): 232–8.
10 Brunk D. Vaginal delivery a risk factor for candidemia. *Ob Gyn News* 2003, Dec 15: 38(24): 14.

CHAPTER 14
ONCE A CAESAREAN ALWAYS A CAESAREAN

1 Craigin EB. Conservatism in obstetrics. *NY Med J* 1916; 104: 1–3.
2 National Institute of Health. *Cesarean Childbirth*. NIH publication no. 82–2067. Government Printing Office, Washington DC 1981.

3 Flamm BL, Newman LA, Thomas ST, Fallon D, Yoshida MM. Vaginal birth after cesarean delivery: Results of a 5-year multicenter collaborative study. *Obstet Gynecol* 1990; 76: 750–4.
4 Rosen MG, Dickinson JC, Westhoff CL. Vaginal birth after cesarean: A meta-analysis of morbidity and mortality. *Obstet Gynecol* 1991; 77: 465–70.
5 Flamm BL, Goings JR, Liu Y, Wolde-Tsadik G. Elective repeat cesarean delivery versus trial of labor: A prospective multicenter study. *Obstet Gynecol* 1994; 83: 927–32.
6 Menacker F, Curtin SC. Trends in cesarean birth and vaginal birth after previous cesarean, 1991–99. *National Vital Statistics Reports* 2001; 49(13): 1–15.
7 *National Vital Statistics Reports* 2003; 51 (11): 1–20.
8 American College of Obstetricians and Gynecologists. *Vaginal Birth After Previous Cesarean Delivery*. Practice Bulletin. ACOG, Washington DC 1999.
9 Troyer LS, Parisi VM. Obstetric parameters affecting success in trial of labor: Designation of a scoring system. *Am J Obstet Gynecol* 1992; 167: 1099–104.
10 Weinstein D, Benshushan A, Tanos V, Zilberstein R, Rojansky N. Predictive score for vaginal birth after cesarean section. *Am J Obstet Gynecol* 1996; 174: 192–8.
11 Troyer LS, Parisi VM. Obstetric parameters affecting success in trial of labor: Designation of a scoring system. *Am J Obstet Gynecol* 1992; 167: 1099–104.
12 Weinstein D, Benshushan A, Tanos V, Zilberstein R, Rojansky N. Predictive score for vaginal birth after cesarean section. *Am J Obstet Gynecol* 1996; 174: 192–8.
13 Flamm BL, Geiger AM. Vaginal birth after cesarean delivery: An admission scoring system. *Obstet Gynecol* 1997; 90: 907–10.
14 Ravasia DJ, Wood SL, Pollard JK. Uterine rupture during induced trial of labor among women with previous cesarean delivery. *Am J Obstet Gynecol* 2000; 183(5): 1176–9.
15 Lydon-Rochelle M, Holt VL, Easterling TR, Martin DP. Risk of uterine rupture during labor among women with prior cesarean delivery. *N Engl J Med* 2001; 345(1): 54–5.
16 Ravasia DJ, Wood SL, Pollard JK. Uterine rupture during induced trial of labor among women with previous cesarean delivery. *Am J Obstet Gynecol* 2000; 183(5): 1176–9.

17 Gregory KD, Korst LM, Cane P, Platt LD, Kahn K. Vaginal birth after cesarean and uterine rupture rates in California. *Obstet Gynecol* 1999; 94: 985–9.

18 Rageth JC, Juzi C, Grossenbacher H. Delivery after previous cesarean: A risk evaluation. *Obstet Gynecol* 1999; 93: 332–7.

19 McMahon MJ, Luther ER, Bowes WA, Olshan AF. Comparison of a trial of labor with an elective second cesarean section. *N Engl J Med* 1996; 335: 689–95.

20 Shipp TD, Zelop C, Repke JT, Cohen A, Caughey AB, Lieberman E. The association of maternal age and symptomatic uterine rupture during a trial of labor after prior cesarean delivery. *Obstet Gynecol* 2002; 99: 585–8.

21 Shipp TD, Zelop C, Cohen A, Repke JT, Lieberman E. Post-cesarean delivery fever and uterine rupture in a subsequent trial of labor. *Obstet Gynecol* 2003; 101: 136–9.

22 Shipp TD, Zelop CM, Repke JT, Cohen A, Lieberman E. Interdelivery interval and risk of symptomatic uterine rupture. *Obstet Gynecol* 2001; 97: 175–7.

23 Chapman SJ, Owen J, Hauth JC. One- versus two-layer closure of a low transverse cesarean: The next pregnancy. *Obstet Gynecol* 1997; 89: 16–18.

24 Bujold E, Bujold C, Hamilton EF, Harel F, Gauthier RJ. The impact of a single-layer or double-layer closure on uterine rupture. *Am J Obstet Gynecol* 2002; 186: 1326–30.

25 Durnwald C, Mercer B. Uterine rupture, perioperative and perinatal morbidity after single-layer and double-layer closure at cesarean delivery. *Am J Obstet Gynecol* 2003; 189: 925–9.

26 Bujold E, Gauthier RJ. Neonatal morbidity associated with uterine rupture: What are the risk factors? *Am J Obstet Gynecol* 2002; 186: 311–14.

27 Smith GCS, Pell JP, Cameron AD, Dobbie R. Risk of perinatal death associated with delivery after previous caesarean section. *JAMA* 2002; 287: 2684–90.

28 Smith GCS, Pell JP, Dobbie R. Caesarean section and risk of unexplained stillbirth in subsequent pregnancy. *Lancet* 2003; 362: 1779–84.

CHAPTER 16
WHAT MOTHERS SAY

1 Clement S. *The Caesarean Experience*. Pandora, London 1991.
2 Moore M, De Costa C. *Cesarean Section*. Johns Hopkins University Press, Baltimore 2003.
3 Wainer Cohen N, Estner L. *Silent Knife*. Bergin and Garvey, Westport CT 1983.
4 Baptisti Richards L. *The Vaginal Birth after Cesarean Experience*. Bergin and Garvey, Westport CT 1987.
5 Odent M. *Birth Reborn*. Pantheon, New York 1984.
6 Donna S. *Baby...Be Born!* Forthcoming.
7 Fisher J, Astbury J, Smith A. Adverse psychological impact of operative obstetrical intervention: a prospective longitudinal study. *Australia New Zealand Journal of Psychiatry* 1997; 31(5): 728–38.

CHAPTER 17
THE PERINEAL PREOCCUPATION

1 Al-Mufti R, McCarthy A, Fisk NM. Obstetricians' personal choice and mode of delivery. *Lancet* 1996; 347: 544.
2 Rortveit G, Dalveit AK, Hannestad YS, Hunskaar S. Urinary incontinence after vaginal delivery or cesarean section. *N Engl J Med* 2003; 348: 900–7.
3 Goldberg RP, Kwon C, Gandhi S, Atkuru LV, Sorensen M, Sand PK. Urinary incontinence among mothers of multiples: the protective effect of cesarean delivery. *Am J Obstet Gynecol* 2003; 188(6): 1447–50.
4 Ryhammer AM, Bek KM, Laurberg S. Multiple vaginal deliveries increase the risk of permanent incontinence of flatus and urine in normal premenopausal women. *Dis Colon Rectum* 1995; 38: 1206–9.
5 MacArthur C, Bick DE, Keigley MRB. Faecal incontinence after childbirth. *Br J Obstet Gynaecol* 1997; 104: 46–50.
6 Sultan AH, Kamm MA, Hudson CN, Bartram CI. Third degree obstetric and anal sphincter tears : risk factors and outcome of primary repair. *BMJ* 1994; 308: 887–91.
7 Dietz HP, Bennett MJ. The effect of childbirth on pelvic organ mobility. *Obstet Gynecol* 2003; 102: 223–8.

8 Neill ME, Swash M. Increased motor unit fibre density in the external anal sphincter muscle in anorectal incontinence: a single EMG study. *J Neurol Neurosurg Psychiat* 1980; 43: 343–7.

9 Sultan AH, Kamm MA, Hudson CN, Thomas JM, Bartram CI. Anal shincter disruption during vaginal delivery. *N Engl J Med* 1993; 329: 1905–11.

10 Fynes M, Donnelly VS, O'Connell PR, O'Herlihy C. Cesarean delivery and anal sphincter injury. *Obstet Gynecol* 1998; 92: 496–500.

11 Odent M. The foetus ejection reflex. *Birth* 1987; 14: 104–5.

12 Odent M. The second stage as a disruption of the foetus ejection reflex. *Midwifery Today*. Autumn 2002: 12.

13 Ferguson JKW. A study of the motility of the intact uterus at term. Surg *Gynecol Obstet* 1941; 73: 359–66.

14 Odent M. Fear of death during labour. *J Reprod Infant Psychol* 1991; 9: 43–7.

15 Newton N, Foshee D, Newton M. Experimental inhibition of labor through environmental disturbance. *Obstet Gynecol* 1967; 371–7.

16 Newton N. The foetus ejection reflex revisited. *Birth* 1987; 14: 106–8.

17 Odent M. *The Scientification of Love*. Free Association Books, London 1999 (revised edition 2001).

CHAPTER 18
EITHER ... OR ...

1 Wilkes PT, Wolf DM, et al. Risk factors for cesarean delivery at presentation of nulliparous patients in labor. *Obstet Gynecol* 2003; 102(6): 1352–7.

2 Odent M. La réflexothérapie lombaire. Efficacité dans le traitement de la colique néphrétique et en analgésie obstétricale. *La Nouvelle Presse Médicale* 1975; 4(3): 188.

3 Odent M. Birth under water. *Lancet* 1983: 1476–7.

4 Norsk P, Epstein M. Effects of water immersion on arginine vasopressin release in humans. *J Appl Physiol* 1988; 64(1): 1–10.

5 Gutkowska J., Antunes-Rodrigues J., McCann Sm. Atrial natriuretic peptide in brain and pituitary gland. *Physiological Reviews* 1997; 77 (2): 465–515, C-2.

6   Mukaddam-Daher S, Jankowski M, et al. Regulation of cardiac oxytocin system and natriuretic peptide during rat gestation and postpartum. *J Endocrinol* 2002; 175(1): 211–16.

7   Gutkowska J, Jankowski M, et al. Oxytocin releases atrial natriuretic peptide by combining with oxytocin receptors in the heart. *Proceedings of the National Academy of Sciences*, USA, 1997; 94: 11704–9.

8   Gilbert RE, Tookey PA. The perinatal mortality and morbidity among babies delivered in water. *BMJ* 1999; 319: 483–7.

9   Rosenear SK, Fox R, Marlow N. Stirrat GM. Birthing pools and the foetus. *Lancet* 1993; 342: 1048–9.

CHAPTER 19
ANTENATAL SCARE

1   Odent M. The nocebo effect in prenatal care. *Primal Heath Research Newsletter* 1994; 2(2).

2   Odent M. Back to the nocebo effect. *Primal Heath Research Newsletter* 1995; 5 (4).

3   Odent M. Antenatal scare. *Primal Heath Research Newsletter* 2000; 7 (4).

4   Thomas P, Golding J, Peters TJ. Delayed antenatal care: does it affect pregnancy outcome? *Soc Sci Med* 1991; 32: 715–23.

5   Douglas KA, Redman CW. Eclampsia in the United Kingdom. *BMJ* 1994; 309: 1395–400.

6   Vintzileos AM, Ananth CV, et al. The impact of prenatal care in the United States on preterm births in the presence or absence of antenatal high-risk conditions. *Am J Obstet Gynecol* 2002; 187: 1254–7.

7   Vintzileos AM, Ananth CV, et al. The impact of prenatal care on postneonatal deaths in the presence or absence of antenatal high-risk conditions. *Am J Obstet Gynecol* 2002; 187: 1258–62.

8   Binstock MA, Wolde-Tsadik G. Alternative prenatal care: impact of reduced visit frequency, focused visits and continuity of care. *J Reprod Med* 1995; 40: 507–12.

9   Sikorski J, Wilson J, et al. A randomised controlled trial comparing two schedules of antenatal visits: the antenatal project. *BMJ* 1996; 312: 546–53.

10 Villar J, Baaqueel H, et al. WHO antenatal care randomized trial for the evaluation of a new model of routine antenatal care. *Lancet* 2001; 357: 1551–64.

11 Wehbeh H, Matthews RP, et al. The effect of recent cocaine use on the progress of labor. *Am J Obstet Gynecol* 1995; 172: 1014–18.

12 Ewigman BG, Crane JP, et al. Effect of prenatal ultrasound screening on perinatal outcome. *N Engl J Med* 1993; 329: 821–7.

13 Bucher HC, Schmidt J G. Does routine ultrasound scanning improve outcome in pregnancy? Meta-analysis of various outcome measures. *BMJ* 1993; 307: 13–7.

14 Larson T, Falck Larson J, et al. Detection of small-for-gestational-age foetuses by ultrasound screening in a high risk population: a randomized controlled study. *Br J Obstet Gynaecol* 1992; 99: 469–74.

15 Secher NJ, Kern Hansen P, et al. A randomized study of foetal abdominal diameter and foetal weight estimation for detection of light-for-gestation infants in low-risk pregnancy. *Br J Obstet Gynaecol* 1987; 94: 105–9.

16 Johnstone FD, Prescott RJ, et al. Clinical and ultrasound prediction of macrosomia in diabetic pregnancy. *Br J Obstet Gynaecol* 1996; 103: 747–54.

17 Steer P, Alam MA, Wadsworth J, Welch A. Relation between maternal haemoglobin concentration and birth weight in different ethnic groups. *BMJ* 1995; 310: 489–91.

18 Valberg LS. Effects of iron, tin, and copper on zinc absorption in humans. *Am J Clin Nutr* 1984; 40: 536–41.

19 Rayman MP, Barlis J, et al. Abnormal iron parameters in the pregnancy syndrome preeclampsia. *Am J Obstet Gynecol* 2002; 187 (2): 412–18.

20 Wen SW, Liu S, Kramer MS, et al. Impact of prenatal glucose screening on the diagnosis of gestational diabetes and on pregnancy outcomes. *Am J Epidemiol* 2000; 152(11): 1009–14.

21 Symonds EM. Aetiology of pre-eclampsia: a review. *J R Soc Med* 1980; 73: 871–5.

22 Naeye EM. Maternal blood pressure and foetal growth. *Am J Obstet Gynecol* 1981; 141: 780–7.

23 Kilpatrick S. Unlike pre-eclampsia, gestational hypertension is not associated with increased neonatal and maternal morbidity except abruptio. SPO abstracts. *Am J Obstet Gynecol* 1995; 419: 376.

24 Curtis S, et al. Pregnancy effects of non-proteinuric gestational hypertension. SPO Abstracts. *Am J Obst Gynecol* 1995; 418: 376.

25 Kenyon SL, Taylor DJ, Tarnow-Mordi W. Broad spectrum antibiotics for spontaneous preterm labour: the ORACLE II randomized trial. *Lancet* 2001; 357: 989–94.

26 Guise JM, Mahon SM, et al. Screening for bacterial vaginosis in pregnancy. *Am J Prev Med* 2001; 20 (suppl 3): 62–72.

27 MRC/RCOG Working party on cervical cerclage. Final report of the Medical Research Council/Royal College of Obstetricians and Gynaecologists multicentre randomized trial of cervical cerclage. *BJOG* 1993; 100: 516–23.

28 Olsen S, Secher NJ. Low consumption of seafood in early pregnancy as a risk factor for preterm delivery: prospective cohort study. *BMJ* 2002; 324: 447.

29 Odent M, McMillan L, Kimmel T. Prenatal care and sea fish. *Eur J Obstet Gynecol Reproduct Biol* 1996; 68: 49–51.

30 Odent M, Colson S, De Reu P. Consumption of seafood and preterm delivery – Encouraging pregnant women to eat sea fish did not show effect. *BMJ* 2002; 324: 1279.

31 Odent M. Preterm delivery. *Lancet* 2003; 361: 436.

32 Odent M. How effective is the accordion method? *Primal Heath Research Newsletter* 2001; 9(2).

33 Zeeman GZ, Hatab M, Twickler DM. Maternal cerebral blood flow changes in pregnancy. *Am J Obstet Gynecol* 2003; 189(4): 968–72.

34 Odent M. *Birth Reborn*. Pantheon, New York 1984.

CHAPTER 20
RECEIVED IDEAS

1 Odent M. Laboring women are not marathon runners. *Midwifery Today* 1994; 31: 23–6.

2 Cram Elsberry C, Shulman J, Moore DS. Nutrition in labour. Paper presented at the International Confederation of Midwives 23rd Congress in Vancouver, 1993.

3 Paterson R, Seath J, Taft P. Wood C. Maternal and foetal concentrations in plasma and urine. *Lancet* 1967; ii: 862–5.

4 Lawrence GF, Brown VA, Parsons RJ. Foetal maternal conse-

quences of high dose glucose infusion during labour. *Br J Obstet Gynaecology* 1982; 89: 27–32.

5 Morley GK, Mooradian AD, Levine AS, Morley J. Mechanism of pain in diabetic peripheral neuropathy. *Am J Med* 1984; 77: 79–82.

6 Kenepp NB, Shelley WC, et al. Foetal and neonatal hazards of maternal hydration with 5 per cent dextrose before caesarean section. *Lancet* 1982; ii: 1150–2.

7 Hazle NR. Hydration in labour: is routine intravenous hydration necessary? *J Nurse-Midwifery* 1986; 31(4): 171–6.

8 Singhi S, Kang EC, Hall JStE. Hazards of maternal hydration with 5 per cent dextrose. *Lancet* 1982; ii: 335–6.

9 Ludka L. Fasting during labour. Paper presented at the International Confederation of Midwives 21st Congress in The Hague, August 1987.

10 DeWees WP. *A Compendious System of Midwifery*. Carey, Lea, and Blanchard, Philadelphia 1833: 188.

11 Odent M. The foetus ejection reflex. *Birth* 1987; 14: 104–5.

12 Odent M. Position in delivery. *Lancet* 1990 (May 12): 1166.

13 Hemminki E, Saaarikoski S. Ambulation and delayed amniotomy in the first stage of labor. *Eur J Obstet Gynecol Reprod Biol* 1983; 15: 129–39.

14 McManus TJ, Calder AA. Upright posture and the efficiency of labour. *Lancet* 1978; 1: 72–4.

15 Bloom SL, McIntire DD, et al. Lack of effect of walking on labor and delivery. *N Engl J Med* 1998; 339: 76–9.

16 Ibid.

17 Sosa R, Kennell J, et al. The effect of a supportive companion on perinatal problems, length of labor, and mother-infant interaction. *N Engl J Med* 1980; 303: 597–600.

18 Kennell J, Klaus M, et al. Continuous emotional support during labor in a US hospital. *JAMA* 1991; 265: 2197–201.

19 Zhang J, Bernasko JW, et al. Continuous labor support from labor attendant for primiparous women : a meta-analysis. *Obstet Gynecol* 1996; 88: 739–44.

20 Lindow SW, Hendricks MS, et al. The effect of emotional support on maternal oxytocin levels in labouring women. *Eur J Obstet Gynecol Reproduct Med* 1998; 79: 127–9.

21 Hodnett ED, Osborn RW. Effects of continuous intrapartum

professional support on childbirth outcomes. *Res Nurs Health* 1989; 12: 289–97.

22 Klaus M, Kennell J, Robertson SS, Sosa R. Effects of social support on maternal and infant morbidity. *BMJ* 1986; 293: 585–7.

23 Keirse MJNC, Enkin M, Lumley J. Social and professional support during labor, in Chalmers I, Enkin M, Keirse MJNC, eds. *Effective Care in Pregnancy and Child Birth*. Oxford University Press, New York 1989; 2: 805–14.

24 Bertsch TD, Nagashima-Whalen L, et al. Labor support by first-time fathers: direct observations. *J Psychosom Obstet Gynecol* 1990; 11: 251–60.

25 Hodnett ED, Lowe NK, et al. Effectiveness of nurses as providers of birth labor support in North American hospitals. *JAMA* 2002; 11: 1373–81.

26 Odent M. Falling asleep and falling in labour, in *The Farmer and the Obstetrician*. Free Association Books, London 2002; ch. 11.

27 Sosa R, Kennell J, et al. The effect of a supportive companion on perinatal problems, length of labor, and mother-infant interaction. *N Engl J Med* 1980; 303: 597–600.

28 Kennell J, Klaus M, et al. Continuous emotional support during labor in a US hospital. *JAMA* 1991; 265: 2197–201.

29 Gordon NP, Walton D, et al. Effects of providing hospital-based doulas in health maintenance organization hospitals. *Obstet Gynecol* 1999; 93(3): 422–6.

30 Hodnett ED, Lowe NK, et al. Effectiveness of nurses as providers of birth labor support in North American hospitals. *JAMA* 2002; 11: 1373–81.

31 Odent M. Why labouring women don't need support. *Mothering* 1996; 80: 46–51.

32 Gelis J. *L'arbre et le fruit*. Fayard, Paris 1984 (the English translation of the title does not refer to the analogy: *History of Childbirth: Fertility, Pregnancy and Birth in early modern Europe*).

33 Didelot. *Instructions pour les sages-femmes*. Nancy 1770.

CHAPTER 22
TOO RATIONAL TO SURVIVE?

1   De Catanzaro D. *Suicide and Self-damaging Behavior: A Sociobiological Perspective.* Academic Press, New York 1981.
2   Voracek M. Risk of suicide in twins. *Lancet* 2003; 327: 1168.
3   Odent M. *The Scientification of Love.* Free Association Books, London 1999 (revised edition 2001).

INDEX